CHILDREN with EPILEPSY

A Parents Guide

Edited by Helen Reisner

WOODBINE HOUSE · 1988

Copyright ©1988 Woodbine House, Inc.

All rights reserved under International and Pan-American Copyright Conventions.
Published in the United States of America by Woodbine House, Inc.

Library of Congress Catalogue Card Number: 87-051319

ISBN: 0-933149-19-0

Cover Illustration & Design: Gary A. Mohrmann
Book Design & Typesetting: Wordscape, Inc., Washington, D.C.

Cataloging-in-Publication Data

Children with epilepsy.

"Cassettes list": p.258
Bibliography: p.239
Includes index.
1. Epilepsy in children—Popular works.
I. Reisner, Helen, 1949–
RJ496.E6C47   1988   618.92'853   87-51319
ISBN 0-933149-19-0 (pbk.)

Manufactured in the United States of America

4 5 6 7 8 9 10

DEDICATION

It is with great hope for the future that this book is dedicated to children with epilepsy, their brothers, sisters, and mostly—parents.

TABLE OF CONTENTS

Acknowledgements

The most important thanks of all go to my family. My husband, Gary, took over endless hours of child care and offered editorial advice and support. I appreciate his infinite patience and objectivity. Our children, Bobby, Emily, and Will, deserve very special recognition for their unconditional love for us and each other. They provided insight into what it's like to have epilepsy and what it's like to live with a brother who has epilepsy.

There have been many people who helped get this book together. I thank you all from the bottom of my heart. I especially thank the parents who sat with me during the evening hours when the kids were asleep, creating the parents statements sections in this book. I am also greatly indebted to the authors for their contributions and commitment to this project. Without them this book would have been impossible.

Everyone associated with this book is honored to thank Dr. Dreifuss for his support of this publication. His wisdom, compassion and sense of humor has sustained the epilepsy movement for many, many years, and his dedication has had a great impact on the quality of life for people with epilepsy.

I extend my warm thanks to Georgia DeGangi, our son's very first occupational therapist, who came to our home and provided us not only with exceptional therapy for him, but a kind ear, sincere support, and our introduction to the world of special needs kids.

The Montgomery County Association for Retarded Citizens has been our source of information and direction from the very first week we moved to Maryland. Even though our son was still a baby, we called them and discovered a resource so diverse that it was able to provide lists of trained babysitters and sponsored special education advocacy courses. Without Lois Geller, Joyce Glenner, and Cory Moore I'm not sure where we'd be today.

Laurie Harris, from the National Capital Area affiliate of the Epilepsy Foundation of America has been remarkably quick to respond to all our needs for information. Thank you.

Bunny Jarrett and Arlene Fingerhut at the Ivymount School in Rockville, Maryland put up with endless phone calls and never wavered in their friendship and support.

I'd like to thank Tracy Gottleib for her professionalism and understanding, Gilbert Johnson for his work on the glossary, Ann Thorward for her help and Jeanne Ludt for her objectivity and encouragement along the way. Zahava Alon has been my example of dedication and excellence. She unknowingly has provided direction.

The Epilepsy Foundation of America in Landover, Maryland has been a source of enthusiastic support as well as a constant resource for technical information. Robyn Ertwine and Anne Exler, in the National Epilepsy Library and Resource Center, have been particularly helpful, as have Sharon Snider and Barbara Elkin. Thank you. Especially deep thanks and appreciation go to Liz Savage for her participation in this book. I reserve a very special thanks for Ann Scherer who has been a wonderful friend throughout this project.

Terry Rosenberg at Woodbine House deserves recognition, acclaim, and high honors for her painstaking, tireless, and thorough work in making this book a book.

I'd like to close with a very special thanks for Karen Stray-Gunderson and her book, *Babies with Down Syndrome: A New Parents Guide.* Due to the feelings aroused by the introduction in that book, I found the inspiration to pursue creating a book about epilepsy that might inspire others to speak up.

FOREWORD

When Helen Reisner asked me to write a foreword for this book, I thought about the most important things I would want to say to parents of a special needs child—in this case, a son or daughter with epilepsy. First and foremost, you need to know that you are not alone! I know only too well the feelings of fear and isolation that can paralyze a family when the child's disability is first diagnosed. We feel lost, cheated, frustrated, and afraid. We are absolutely certain that we are the only parents who have ever gone through this experience, the only ones who could possibly understand and make sense of the welter of conflicting emotions constantly bombarding us as we seek to understand and cope with our new circumstances.

However, nothing could be further from the truth. Countless parents throughout the country have worked through the tangle of emotions engendered daily by the presence of a child with special needs, and have come to realize and embrace the particularly poignant joys and challenges of raising this child who, after all, is not so very different from his or her nondisabled siblings and peers. And in realizing these truths, these loving, committed people have come to recognize the validity of the old saying about "strength in numbers." Hence the phenomenal growth of the parent support group movement in this country. You, as parents of a child or children with epilepsy, can draw upon the tremendous resources of these support groups, which will enable you to become effective advocates for your children. In order to exert an ultimate positive effect on your child's quality of life, you must be willing to fight for the best, most appropriate medical, educational, and related services, and to work tirelessly to diminish the old, counterproductive and negative stereotypes still plaguing children and adolescents with epilepsy. Although this struggle at times may be difficult, the rewards are boundless and far outweigh the efforts involved.

CHILDREN WITH EPILEPSY: A PARENTS GUIDE provides useful information to aid parents in this struggle. Its ten chapters, written by various professionals and specialists in the field of epilepsy services and disability management, cover all aspects of the disability, with major emphasis on assisting parents and family members to cope with the daily ramifications of epilepsy. In keeping with the book's focus on parental support, the author includes a parent perspective section at the end of each chapter.

It has often been said that "a grief shared is half a grief, but a joy shared is twice a joy." By sharing our grief, as well as our joys, we can find the strength to give our children with special needs the same range of opportunities that all children so richly deserve.

In looking back over my experiences in raising my own special needs daughter, I have often drawn comfort and profound peace of mind from the following prayer: "God grant me the serenity to accept the things I cannot change; the courage to change the things I can; and the wisdom to know the difference."

Patricia McGill Smith *
Deputy Assistant Secretary
Office of Special Education and Rehabilitative Services
United States Department of Education

---

* This foreword was written by Patricia McGill Smith in her private capacity. No official support or endorsement of this book by the U.S. Department of Education is intended or should be inferred.

INTRODUCTION

Helen and Gary Reisner

When we saw our son's first seizure, he was just three months old. At first we weren't even sure it was a seizure. It looked like an exaggerated moro reflex. We kept wondering what it could be, but didn't have the knowledge to make any real diagnosis. We were really scared.

We watched Will seize for the next few days while trying to convince our pediatrician something was wrong. When the doctor finally saw our son have a seizure, we asked him if it could be epilepsy. He told us it was a seizure disorder, that the word epilepsy wasn't used anymore.

That visit to the pediatrician was the beginning of our search for accurate and up-to-date information. We wanted to know the difference between epilepsy and seizure disorder and we knew little about either one. It turned out that our son's epilepsy was a syndrome called infantile spasms and we couldn't find much at all to read except for some grim medical textbooks. We were in a dark tunnel, with truly not a flicker of light at the other end.

So many parents feel, as we do, that having a child with epilepsy is living in the unknown. Neurologists, through no fault of their own, simply cannot answer many of our most important questions. It is difficult to predict what path most epilepsies will take. It makes it impossible to work within a range of expectations.

The adjustment to epilepsy and to having a child who has special needs, has been heart-wrenching, disruptive, painful, traumatic, shattering; you name it. It is simply downright awful. Although we have had a tough battle adjusting to Will's handicap, we did accept right away that we could not turn back, we could not rewrite our son's destiny. We realized that we had the power to provide the best possible medical, educational, and social experiences for him, but we could not fix him. We could not make the seizures go away. So we went on from there.

We began the process of trying to educate ourselves and in so doing realized how vital it is for all parents to learn everything they can about what is happening to their children. The more informed you become about the various seizure types, especially the type your child has, the more information you will be able to share with others. This is important, particularly for the people responsible for your child's care and education and it is essential for you as you try to manage your child's illness.

Since we had difficulty finding books about epilepsy, we had the feeling that there was a book that should be written. As we became involved with other parents, it became even clearer. We began thinking more and more about what kind of information parents of children with epilepsy need.

We have attempted to give you insight and direction, but have learned through our own experience that epilepsy is an illness that requires learning new information as your child's epilepsy changes or evolved. There really is no one book that will answer all your questions.

There are many resources beyond this book to help you. The Reading List in the back of this book is the logical next step in your study of epilepsy. Get on the phone and call for help, ideas, advice counseling, and contact with other parents. No source of information is as meaningful as that from other parents who have been through it.

In your studies you will discover that the language of epilepsy is new and confusing. It might surprise you that it is also new and confusing to medical and educational professionals. As advances in research have led to a better understanding of epilepsy, and new drugs and treatments have been developed, a new and precise vocabulary evolved. In fact, during the last ten years major steps have been taken to clearly define the different seizures so that there could be a universal understanding. It is for this reason that you may hear "grand mal" instead of "tonic clonic;" "petit mal" instead of "absence;" "psychomotor" instead of "complex partial". The list of changes is too long to go on here, however, we urge you to refer to the Glossary. If you hear an unfamiliar term, *never* jump to the conclusion that you are uninformed, ask for an explanation. A very common question in the field of epilepsy is, "What does that mean?"

We hope that this book will help you learn about epilepsy, your child's experience, and help your family adjust to a diagnosis that in years past was far more devastating than today. Due to families working to increase public awareness and understanding, there is a new world for our children full of opportunity. Children with epilepsy need not bear an outdated burden of shame, misunderstanding, or fear. As parents we must see to it that they do not.

ONE

What Is Epilepsy?

FRITZ E. DREIFUSS, M.B., F.R.C.P., F.R.A.C.P.*

Epilepsy, with its mixture of physical and psychic symptoms, has long held a significant position in the struggle between science and magic. For centuries the prevailing belief was that epilepsy was a manifestation of demonic possession inflicted on people who had sinned against one or another deity. Scientists struggled against this tide of superstition toward a more factual explanation for epilepsy. In 175 A.D., Galen not only recognized that it was a disease of the brain, but actually separated the epilepsies as those that were of unknown cause, and those that were a result of other diseases.

At the end of the nineteenth century, Hughlings Jackson and Gowers ushered in a new era with their astute observations and critical evaluations. Jackson recognized that epilepsy consisted of different kinds of temporary disorders of function – sensory as well as motor – and mental as well as physical. And he recognized that epilepsy consisted of an electrical discharge in the nerve cells of the brain.

As scientific research continues into the physical causes and treatments of epilepsy, one of the primary tasks remains educating people about epilepsy and banishing forever the misunderstanding attached to this disorder. In order to do that, parents need to become better informed themselves as to what epilepsy is. I have written this chapter

---

* Fritz E. Dreifuss is a Professor of Neurology, School of Medicine, University of Virginia and Director of the Comprehensive Epilepsy Program in Charlottesville, Virginia.

1

as a beginning source for you. I urge you to read further, ask questions, and become involved with your child's treatment.

Definition of Epilepsy

Epilepsy is a condition where recurrent electrical discharges in the brain disturb the normal functioning of the nervous system. These episodes of disturbance are called *seizures*. Seizures can involve a temporary loss of consciousness or temporary changes in behavior. The exact changes of behavior depend on the area of the brain which is being stimulated by the electrical discharge.

Causes of Epilepsy

The brain consists of 14,000 million nerve cells, many of which are connected by little junctions through which electrical impulses are sent from one to another by means of chemical substances known as *neurotransmitters*. An electrical impulse releases the neurotransmitters which then activate the next nerve cell. These electrical impulses fire in regular patterns called *brain waves*. When many of these nerve cells fire abnormally at the same time, an epileptic seizure may result.

The sudden excessive firing of nerve cells in the brain is like an electrical storm and the seizure itself is the way the body physically reacts to this storm. When the seizure is over, the storm may clear suddenly or the affected nerve cells may be so exhausted as to require a rest period, which accounts for the prolonged period of confusion or sleepiness that may follow a seizure.

There are many reasons seizures occur. One of these is an instability of the brain cells which is caused by trauma, scars, chemical causes, inflammation, tumor, intoxication, or malformations. Another reason is an imbalance between neurotransmitters. Epilepsy in itself is usually not a disease but a symptom which may come about as a result of different causes, just as a headache may be a symptom of different conditions.

About half of all epileptic seizures have an identifiable cause and we call those seizures *symptomatic* or *secondary*. The other half are thought to have a genetically determined metabolic cause and here the seizures are known as *idiopathic* or *primary*. In children, the idiopathic causes outnumber the symptomatic and in adults the opposite is true.

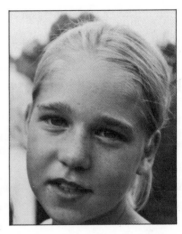

There are many different causes of symptomatic epilepsy including a scar, a tumor, a loss of blood supply, certain toxins, certain metabolic products from abnormal metabolism, a lack of blood sugar, or a lack of calcium. The brain only responds to these different causes in one of two ways. It either stops functioning, in which case there is paralysis, or it has seizures.

In the idiopathic or primary epilepsies, there is a genetically inherited tendency to epilepsy, *not* the epilepsy itself. Environmental factors, such as sleep deprivation and flickering lights can trigger seizures in someone who is genetically susceptible.

Classification of Seizures

There are many different types of seizures. It is very important to classify them so that the proper drugs can be prescribed. Also, classification enables physicians to exchange information, and this communication is essential for advances in knowledge. The International Classification now in use defines the following types of seizures:

Generalized Seizures

During a generalized seizure, the epileptic discharge affects the brain as a whole. It probably begins in a deep central structure and spreads throughout the brain on both sides. The signal symptom is nearly always loss of consciousness. There are four major types of generalized seizures that affect children. They include:

Absence Seizures. During an absence seizure, the brain's normal activity shuts down. The child stares blankly, sometimes rotates his eyes upward, and occasionally blinks or jerks repetitively, he drops objects from his hand, and there may be some mild involuntary movements known as *automatisms*. The attack lasts for a few seconds and then it is over as rapidly as it began. If these attacks occur dozens of times each day, they can interfere with your child's school performance and be confused by parents and teachers with daydreaming.

Myoclonic Seizures. Here there is a sudden jerk which may be relatively mild and confined to individual muscle groups or may be a massive jerk which can throw your child to the ground. While absence seizures usually signify a relatively benign form of epilepsy, myoclonic jerks frequently are associated with more severe and progressively worsening conditions.

Atonic or Drop Attacks. These are characterized by a sudden slumping of the whole body due to a loss of muscle tone and an inability to stay in an upright position. They are relatively rare and are frequently associated with rather severe and progressive forms of epilepsies, although they may be seen in less severe conditions. This is the type of seizure that leads to facial and head injuries; headgear is recommended.

Tonic/Clonic Seizures. These represent what used to be called the *grand mal* convulsion in which your child falls to the ground, sometimes after a loud cry. His body becomes rigid in the tonic phase, then begins to jerk during the clonic phase. After several seconds to several minutes, he may fall into a deep sleep or be temporarily confused. Your child may bite his tongue, but these bites are not usually serious and heal rapidly. Your child may lose bladder control during a seizure. After the seizure, he may complain of muscle soreness or headache.

Partial (Focal, Local) Seizures

Unlike generalized seizures, which affect the brain as a whole, partial seizures remain confined to circumscribed areas of the brain. Here the symptoms depend on the area of the brain involved in the seizure.

Simple Partial Seizures. During simple partial seizures, the person remains conscious. The seizure may cause a body part, for example a leg, to jerk. This may spread to other parts of the same side of the body. This type of seizure is the result of an abnormal discharge affecting those nerve cells which are responsible for movement. A seizure in the sensory portion of the brain will produce abnormal sensory sensations. If the visual part of the brain is involved, abnormal visual phenomena can occur, such as vivid scenes, or nonexistent objects. If the temporal lobe is involved, abnormal psychic sensations, including feelings of unreality or memory disturbances, will occur. This seizure type may trigger feelings of fear, anger, or excitement.

Complex Partial Seizures. These are like simple partial seizures except that the discharge spreads into the areas of the brain responsible for keeping a person conscious. During a complex partial seizure, consciousness will be disturbed, or lost. A complex partial seizure may be the result of a simple partial seizure that spreads into those areas determining consciousness. During these attacks, there may be automatisms in which the person engages in abnormal but possibly purposeful-appearing activity, such as pulling at or fumbling with his clothes, chewing, or lip smacking, which he cannot recall after he regains consciousness.

Regardless of whether the person has simple partial seizures or complex partial seizures, seizures may spread to involve the whole brain, at which time consciousness will be lost and a generalized tonic/clonic seizure may occur. This is known as a *secondarily generalized seizure;* that is, one which begins in one specific location and then becomes generalized.

Status Epilepticus

This occurs when seizures follow one upon the next without the person regaining consciousness between attacks. If the seizures are generalized tonic/clonic seizures, then the status epilepticus is a life-threatening event. If they are absence seizures they have considerably less grave implications. If status epilepticus involves partial seizures, such as partial motor seizures, we call it *continuous partial epilepsy.*

What To Do When Your Child Has a Seizure

1. Leave your child where he is *unless* he is in danger of hurting himself by banging his head against an object.
2. Do not put any object into your child's mouth. It is anatomically impossible for him to swallow his tongue. You can do more damage by possibly breaking one of his teeth or causing damage to his lungs.
3. If he is wearing tight clothing, loosen it.

4. Turn your child on his side so that he does not inhale mucus or blood.
5. If the seizure lasts longer than five minutes, call an ambulance·

Some of the Consequences of Seizures

Neurological Consequences

Epileptic seizures may cause brain cell changes. In severe and prolonged seizures, energy requirements may not be met because of greatly excessive demand, and a lack of enough oxygen to meet that demand. Low blood pressure and metabolic changes may cause further trouble.

These neurological consequences have either subtle or obvious consequences depending on the severity of the injury to the brain. Epileptic seizures may interfere with intellectual functioning and perhaps even cause developmental delays. They can also cause physical handicaps. That is not to say that every seizure is followed by these drastic consequences, but severe recurrent seizures or very prolonged seizures carry with them the potential for neurological consequences. There is, however, no reliable evidence that absence seizures or isolated short tonic/clonic seizures cause damage.

Psychological Consequences

Seizures can result in a wide variety of psychological consequences. Social, educational, and vocational handicaps should not be allowed to develop since they can impair your child's ability to function. The exact handicaps will vary from child to child. The psychological consequences to your child are covered more fully in later chapters.

Kindling

There is some evidence that untreated or uncontrolled seizures predispose the brain to more seizures. In other words, the brain learns epilepsy by the setting up of epileptic circuits if subsequent seizures are not prevented. Thus, it is possible that seizures carry within themselves the seeds of future seizures. It is the same process as learning itself. In learning, the recurrent use of certain circuits imprint upon the brain the information given it. The brain sets up circuits in response to incoming information. If that incoming information is an abnormal electrical discharge, this circuitry becomes ingrained in the brain and connections develop to keep that circuit going. This is known as *kindling*.

Epileptic Syndromes

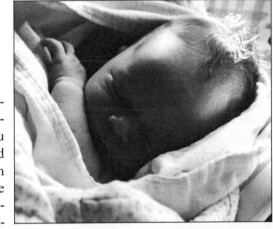

Epileptic seizures are the symptoms that lead you to take your child to a physician. In many cases these symptoms represent a specific syndrome which includes not only the seizure but also the condition causing the seizure. Sometimes the syndromes causing the seizures are benign and require only short-term treatment. Other times they indicate a severe and occasionally progressive condition. Epileptic syndromes are frequently age-related.

If your child is a newborn, his *neonatal seizures* are frequently symptoms of severe brain insult, including prenatal infections, malformations, the complications of prematurity, the results of deprivation of oxygen and blood supply, and occasionally severe metabolic disorders. In the group of prenatal and natal insults, the outlook is quite poor. A high percentage of such infants develop serious neurological problems.

Infantile Spasms are a severe form of epilepsy. It covers a variety of conditions with different outlooks. It is important to recognize infantile spasms early. This is not always easy, but early diagnosis and intervention can contribute to therapeutic success.

In the idiopathic variety of infantile spasms, the condition begins between the ages of three and six months, after previously normal development. Treatment with ACTH is frequently successful. The seizures are characterized by sudden myoclonic jerks with flexing of the neck and body and stiffening of the limbs. These are very short seizures frequently occurring in clusters. The outlook for neurological and intellectual development is frequently satisfactory.

In the symptomatic form, the age of onset is earlier, neurologic development is frequently abnormal, and the success of therapy is less predictable. The outlook is grave and more severe seizures of the Lennox-Gastaut syndrome often occur.

Lennox-Gastaut Syndrome is a blanket term covering a variety of seizures including atonic drop attacks, complex partial seizures, absence seizures, and occasionally tonic/clonic seizures. This is an extremely difficult condition to treat, is often associated with significant delay in motor and intellectual development, and does not respond very well to drugs. It is probably the end result of a variety of underlying conditions.

As in the case of infantile spasms, Lennox-Gastaut syndrome covers a variety of conditions with different outlooks. In some cases, the outlook is not at all bad. The seizures may be relatively self-limited, relatively easy to control with a single drug, and the child's intellectual function relatively intact, although he may be a little slower in intellectual development than would be expected. However, Lennox-Gastaut syndrome also is seen in a very severe form where the condition is part of a more significant underlying brain disturbance. When this occurs, the outlook is much worse, both in intellectual development and in ultimate control of seizures. It is here that a variety of drugs is tried and if these drugs fail, a ketogenic diet is tried.

It must be emphasized that the outlook varies according to the nature of the underlying brain disturbance. When no underlying brain disease is evident–called idiopathic or primary epilepsy–the outlook is very much more favorable than when the epilepsy is only one manifestation of a severe brain disturbance. In the case of a severe brain disturbance, even the ultimate control of these seizures will not result in normal development.

Rolandic Epilepsy is a syndrome with a much better prognosis. It is also referred to as a benign partial seizure of childhood or *ideopathic partial seizure*. It occurs in the first ten years of life and is characterized by partial motor seizures, usually occurring at night. Generally, it responds very well to most drugs. The condition usually goes away during a child's adolescence. The child usually has no underlying neurological disturbance, the outlook is extremely favorable, and the risk of severe seizures is very small.

Pyknoleptic Petit Mal is a syndrome of childhood absence seizures with an extremely good outlook. Seizures consist of absence attacks occurring as often as a hundred times a day. It responds well to valproate and ethosuximide and tends to disappear around puberty. Exercise, hyperventilation, and drowsiness can cause these seizures.

Juvenile Myoclonic Epilepsy is a syndrome characterized by generalized tonic/clonic seizures, usually near the time of awakening in the morning. Frequently there is a history of absence seizures and myoclonic jerks. This epilepsy responds extremely well to valproate, but it is a good idea to avoid deprivation and flashing lights since these can cause attacks.

Febrile Seizures

Febrile seizures are associated with a fever. They are quite common. At some time they may affect as much as 3 to 5 percent of the population. Almost half of the people have recurrent febrile seizures, but only about 3 to 5 percent develop epilepsy.

As with the epileptic syndromes, there is more than one variety of febrile seizure. *Benign febrile seizures* occur in normal children without neurological disturbance, often with a strong family history of similar seizures where the attacks are relatively short and simple. They usually occur near the beginning of an illness.

Another variety frequently occurs in children who have neurological handicaps. In this case, the seizures may last longer, appear in clusters, and may be focal. If your child has this variety, together with an abnormal electroencephalogram (EEG), then he may be at risk to develop epilepsy later.

Simple febrile seizures often require no treatment, but if recurrences are frequent, intermittent therapy with diazepam or long-term preventive therapy with phenobarbital might be considered.

Diagnosis

In epilepsy a diagnosis is critical. Because particular seizure types respond to particular drugs better than to others, the classification of seizures is now of more than theoretical importance. An accurate history from patients and observers and, if necessary, the recording of seizures with appropriate EEG verification is of greater importance than ever in order to design the most appropriate treatment plan. This section reviews how a diagnosis is made.

Clinical History

One of the most important features of an examination is the *clinical history*, which is a record of all previous events, including the mother's pregnancy, the child's birth, early development, the history of any illnesses or hospitalizations, and a very detailed account of the onset and the course of the condition. For example, it is critical to know whether a particular incident preceded the onset of the seizures, or whether there was an associated fever, ear infection, head trauma, or other potential cause. A careful description of the nature of the attacks is necessary in order to make a diagnosis of the type of seizures and the type of epilepsy under consideration. Frequency and time relationships, such as clustering of seizures, may be important. The duration of the seizures and a careful description of events during and after the seizures are also important. A complete family history is necessary because inherited conditions may cause seizures.

The Physical Examination

The *physical examination* and the *neurological examination* produce evidence of any disease of the nervous system or other body parts. Tests include studies of the blood, particularly blood chemistries such as sugar, calcium, and abnormal constituents. An EEG is performed to help confirm the diagnosis of epilepsy and indicate which part of the brain is particularly involved. Remember, however, that a certain number of people with epilepsy will still have normal EEGs on occasion. The *CT scan*, which is a sophisticated radiological test, produces pictures of the nervous system and abnormalities of blood flow and blood vessels. Scars and tumors may frequently be seen in this way. The magnetic resonance image, or *MRI scan*, is a computer-assembled picture that results in an even sharper image of the brain. In a few cases, the evaluation may require a *PET scan*. This stands for Positron Emission Tomography, and identifies the metabolic activities of various areas of the nervous system and changes which may indicate where the seizure focus is located. Obviously, not every person with epilepsy requires all or even a majority of these tests.

Treatment

Once your child has been diagnosed, and his physician and you have decided on a course of treatment, certain treatment principles should be observed.

First, the specific antiepileptic drug should be chosen after evaluating the risk-benefit proportions for your child. This involves you and the physician reviewing what the drug will do to help eliminate seizures and what its side effects are. Once the drug of choice has been established, you and your child (if he is old enough) should be edu-

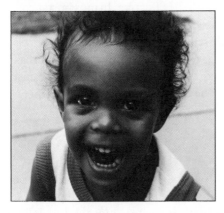

cated in its use, its potential side effects, and the necessity for regular administration.

Although seizure control is the main aim of your child's treatment, it is wise to make sure the dose regimen is within the recognized therapeutic range. Sometimes, a child is in danger of being overdosed in order to eliminate his seizures.

At first your child should only be given one drug and he should take it long enough for your physician to be able to judge its effect. He will have serum blood levels taken frequently until the situation has stabilized, after which blood levels can be taken less frequently, sometimes only once a year.

Blood Levels

Analyzing blood for the antiepileptic drug level will tell your physician the amount of medication in your child's body. He needs that information to determine if your child is receiving adequate doses of medication. The drug is absorbed and coats the cells in the brain. The level in the blood slowly reaches a point where the coating action is constant. This is referred to as *steady state*. The steady state is maintained by taking medications and is monitored by blood samples to see if the medication has reached the *therapeutic blood level*.

If your child misses a dose of his medication, it will effect this blood level. Call your physician immediately to find out if, or when, you should give the missed dose.

The therapeutic blood level range is that quantity of drug in the blood which usually controls seizures without producing undue side-effects. Higher blood levels are more likely to be associated with side-effects. This is called a *toxic* level and seizures are likely to break through. When blood levels are too low—this is called *below therapeutic*—the drug is likely to be ineffective and seizures can break through. Individuals vary and some require higher levels than the so-called therapeutic range for the drug to be effective. In most instances, blood levels are monitored during the early stages of treatment and at variable intervals thereafter. Most physicians will get blood levels when signs of an overdose appear or if seizures unexpectedly break through. Sometimes other blood tests are given to guard against depression of the blood count or the development of abnormal metabolic effects such as liver abnormalities.

Drug Side Effects

Almost all drugs have side effects. However, not all children taking a particular drug develop those side effects. With antiepileptics, the side effects are usually evident early in the treatment and are mild. It is a peculiarity of antiepileptic drugs that some children respond well and others do not. That is why it is important that you be aware of the potential side effects of any drug your child is taking. Take time to learn all about your child's medication. Ask the doctor for all the possible side effects so you know what to look for. Your child is an individual and you are in the best possible position to observe what his individual reaction will be to any medication. Follow your instincts and let your physician know if you suspect anything unusual. If is far better to err on the side of caution than to "let it wait" just one more day.

Often parents tend to blame their child's medication for any changes in the child's behavior. Usually, however, these behaviors are the result of the same impairment that is causing your child to have epilepsy. Antiepileptic drugs do not generally cause behavior and learning problems.

Drug Interactions

If your child's seizures have not been controlled and his blood levels have been in the therapeutic range, either a change in his drug or the addition of a second drug should be considered. If he is taking more than one drug, your physician should be knowledgeable about how the drugs interact.

At one time, multiple antiepileptic drugs were administered simultaneously in the belief that they were more effective and there were no additional side effects. It is now realized that most patients with seizures will respond just as well to one drug as to a mixture, and that multiple drugs interacting with each other complicates treatment. In addition, the side effects do increase, particularly those which reduce alertness, increase depression, anxiety, and fatigue, and interfere with cognitive function. The administration of one drug, called *monotherapy*, leads to increased alertness and therefore a better quality of life *even though the seizure frequency does not necessarily decrease*.

In some instances, drug interactions will increase the amount of medication in your child's system and at other times decrease them. For example, when valproic acid and phenobarbital are given simultaneously, metabolic interaction increases the amount of phenobarbital in the blood. Other factors, such as illness, affect the metabolism of antiepileptic drugs and cause changes in blood levels which may or may not be predictable, leading to the necessity for more frequent blood tests.

Many factors besides drug interactions may influence the frequency of seizures and they must all be taken into account when more than one drug is prescribed. These factors include hormonal changes that may occur around the time of the menstrual period, and they may also be noted during puberty. Changes in hormonal concentrations may alter the metabolism of antiepileptic drugs and change the body's requirement. This is particularly true in puberty when the rapid meta-

Figure 1. Commonly Used Antiepileptics

Drug	Trade Name	Usual Dose (mg/kg/day)	Therapeutic Range (µg/mL)	Side Effects
Carba-mazepine	Tegretol	10–15	5–12	drowsiness, dizziness, blurred vision, lethargy, nausea, vomiting, possible blood cell depression.
Phenytoin	Dilantin	5–10	10–20	confusion, blurred speech, nausea, increased growth of body hair, gum overgrowth, tremor, anemia, loss of coordination, double vision.
Phenobarbital	Luminal	4–6	15–40	drowsiness, lethargy, hyperactivity, loss of learning ability.
Primidone	Mysoline	12–25	5–10	vomiting, dizziness, loss of coordination, drowsiness, appetite loss, irritability, nausea.
Ethosuximide	Zarontin	15–35	40–100	drowsiness, nausea, vomiting, sleep disturbance, hiccups.
Valproic Acid	Depakene/ Depakote	15–60	50–100	hair loss, tremor, possible liver damage, pancreatitis, nausea, vomiting, indigestion, sedation.
Clonazepam	Clonopin	0.05–0.2	20–80 (ng/mL)	lethargy, dizziness, increased salivation, increase in bronchial secretions.

bolism of childhood gives way to the adult style. Other factors include emotional stress and illness, including fevers, which may increase the likelihood of seizures. Drugs such as antibiotics, antihistamines, antipsychotic drugs, and antiasthma drugs may change the threshold for seizures or may interact with the antiepileptic drugs. Figure 1 lists the commonly used antiepileptic drugs. It is best to ask your physician to explain in detail which drugs interact.

Length of Treatment

There are no hard and fast rules about the duration of therapy after seizures are controlled. Some types of seizures, such as absence and benign childhood seizures, go into remission during adolescence.

Seizures which have as their basis an underlying brain lesion are more likely to continue indefinitely, although even there, as the brain matures, the seizures become less frequent. Discontinuation of medication might be considered after a seizure-free period of several years. Many physicians recommend a seizure-free period of two to four years, and a normal EEG before considering discontinuation of medications. I feel that each patient should be treated individually. For example, if at the end of the seizure-free period the person is a child, I discontinue medication with more confidence than if the patient is a teenager about to get a driver's license, about to start dating, or about to leave home to live in a college dormitory. In any event, the individual should participate in the decision-making process and should be told the potential risks of stopping the medication. If medications are discontinued, they are usually tapered off over several months, rather than discontinued suddenly.

People do not generally "outgrow" epilepsy, but in some epileptic syndromes, particularly those of primary epilepsy, and the pyknoleptic petit mal syndrome of absence seizures, there is a tendency to spontaneous remission around puberty. Even so, these people will have a rather lower threshold for a recurrence of seizures under conditions of stress such as sleep deprivation and the administration of certain drugs, including alcohol. Most epilepsies are not outgrown in the same way as epilepsy is not cured but only controlled. On the other hand, when a person has remained seizure-free for an appropriate time, cautious withdrawal of medication may be in the person's best interest.

Other Treatment Methods

In a very few children, *surgery* is indicated. If your child has uncontrolled seizures, your physician may be considering surgery for him. However, of the 20 percent of people with epilepsy who have uncontrolled seizures, only a very small percentage are even candidates for surgery. In order for your child to be considered for surgery, his seizures must be:

1. Focal in origin.
2. Occur in one part of the brain, on one side.

3. In an area that does not control important functions such as speech, or motor control.

When evaluating the prospects of surgery, keep in mind that new drugs are always being researched and there is the possibility of a new drug to help your child. Also, seizures often become less severe and frequent as a child gets older.

Surgery is performed for one of three reasons. Either to remove lesions resulting from injury or disease, to remove the portion of the brain where the seizures occur, or to remove a portion of the brain to prevent the seizures from spreading. This last reason is similar to the plan where you cut down some of the trees surrounding a forest fire in order to prevent the fire from spreading.

If you are considering surgery, the Epilepsy Foundation of America has a list of doctors and/or centers experienced in these procedures. It would be a good idea to contact them and see what doctors and facilities are available in your area and discuss these with your physician.

In some very intractable types of early childhood epilepsy, a *ketogenic diet* may occasionally be used. In these cases, your child's diet is modified so that it consists mainly of fat, with relatively little protein and virtually no carbohydrates. Because of the need to include a necessary number of calories, such a diet is difficult to prepare, particularly as most fat diets are quite unpalatable. Occasionally drop attacks, myoclonic seizures, and other convulsive phenomena may respond to such a diet. You can only continue a ketogenic diet for a limited time because your child needs other nutrients. Since the introduction of valproate, the ketogenic diet has been used less often.

Sometimes when seizures are precipitated by predictable stress factors, *relaxation, exercises,* and *biofeedback* may be beneficial. These have to be used together with other more standard treatments, including antiepileptic drugs. *Vitamins* and *food supplements* should be given as a treatment only where there are diseases which are the result of deficiencies, either in your child's diet or in his metabolism. Food fads, megavitamins, and elimination diets have no place in the treatment of epilepsy unless there are specific indications for the use of such treatments for other health reasons.

Unfortunately, wherever there is a chronic condition causing hardship, there will develop untested claimed "cures." The history of epilepsy is filled with these, including the wearing of garlic around the neck, amulets, and copper bracelets. Unscientific treatments have ranged from purging to bloodletting. Do not be taken in by untested or foolish treatments.

Goals of Treatment

The Elimination of Seizures

Since seizures are symptoms of a brain disturbance, the most effective means of eliminating seizures are those which eliminate the underlying cause. Some epileptic seizures cause damage to the brain by greatly exceeding the ability of the system to keep the nerve cells functioning, thereby depriving them of oxygen. Seizures can also cause physical, social, psychological, vocational, and recreational impairment, thereby irreversibly altering a person's quality of life and ability to cope.

The majority of cases of epilepsy will have to be treated by working on the symptoms not the causes. This generally means the use of antiepileptic drugs. To some extent, treatment will depend on the nature, the severity, the frequency, and the predictability of seizures. For example, isolated sleep seizures, reflex-precipitated epilepsy, and self-limited childhood seizures have different treatments than frequent bouts of status epilepticus and episodes associated with prolonged periods of confusion.

Prevention

Obviously we want to prevent epilepsy from occurring whenever we can. One way is to try to prevent such epilepsy-causing events as head injuries, brain infections, inflammatory illnesses, and early teenage pregnancies. It is possible that the development of epilepsy can be prevented by using antiepileptic drugs after head injuries and in the case of recurrent febrile seizures.

We also want to prevent seizures. We can do this with drugs or surgery and by avoiding or eliminating precipitating factors such as alcohol, sleep deprivation, and other factors known to trigger seizures.

Whatever means of therapy we choose, a major goal should be to achieve the best possible outcome at the least possible cost to you and your child. This includes costs as measured in:

1. Cerebral damage from surgery. While surgery may curb seizures, it may be prohibitive in terms of the amount of neurological damage.
2. Drug toxicity may make your child unable to function effectively as a result of intolerable side effects.
3. Expense may be a major consideration. Occasionally a compromise may have to be made between the best possible medication regimen and that which is economically possible. Such a compromise may make the difference between acceptable seizure control and no treatment at all.

The Hospital

Generally there is no need to take your child to a hospital unless his seizure lasts longer than ten minutes or there is a rapid succession of overlapping seizures which, in the case of generalized tonic/clonic seizures, may be life threatening and, in the case of partial seizures, though less severe, may also require attention.

When a person with recurrent seizures (status epilepticus) goes to the emergency room, he will be placed flat on a bed with padded side rails. A physician may insert a tube to ensure that the breathing passages are not obstructed or administer oxygen if the person is blue. Usually an intravenous fluid to administer medicine is started. The medication usually begins with a drug such as diazepam (Valium) and continues with a longer-acting drug such as phenytoin (Dilantin). General anesthesia is only used when other measures fail to control seizures.

Treating the Whole Child

Every seizure disorder threatens your child's ability to cope physically and emotionally. His coping style is determined by his age, the site of the responsible lesion, the side of the brain in which seizures occur, the nature and dose of medications, as well as his underlying personality, family support systems, and ability to handle stress. All these factors must be considered in your child's overall treatment program, which consists of very much more than just administering medication and evaluating drug levels. The participation of social workers, educational consultants, and vocational rehabilitation counselors adds immeasurably to the quality of his lifestyle and may also directly influence the degree of seizure control. In every instance, a community resource person who is familiar with all the professional and voluntary resources available to you should be a member of the treatment team.

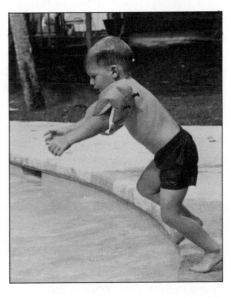

If the right treatment team is not available and your child has not responded rapidly to medical therapy, he may be referred to an epilepsy unit, where such resources are available. These epilepsy programs have the capability for intensive monitoring and a multidisciplinary approach using the above treatment resources.

Parents' desire to shield their children from potential harm is great. In the case of a child with epilepsy, however, protectiveness very easily leads to overprotectiveness. This prevents him from engaging in activities which are necessary for him to become an independent, confident adult. However, some restrictions are necessary, including not driving until a certain seizure-free interval has passed. No one with a history of seizures should operate an aircraft or a commercial passenger vehicle. People with epilepsy should not bathe by themselves, as drowning is not uncommon under these circumstances, particularly since immersion in water sometimes triggers seizures. This prohibition does not extend to supervised sports, including swimming. I do not favor the sports in which head injury is a frequent consequence, particularly boxing, but am opposed to this sport for anyone, since its very essence is an attempt to cause a head injury. Playing football is still an open question. Probably most people with epilepsy whose seizures are well-controlled can play football, but if the seizures are the consequence of head injury in the first place, this sport should also be restricted.

Epilepsy education should form part of every treatment program and should be aimed at everyone your child is likely to come in contact with, from family, to school, and to the public in general. Professional education aimed at school nurses, medical students, pediatricians, and family practitioners should be a part of a strong advocacy group with a chapter organization like the Epilepsy Foundation of America. These groups can do much to influence attitudes about epilepsy.

Noncompliance

The most common cause for poor seizure control is not following the physician's directions in taking the prescribed medication. This is known as *noncompliance*. A person can be noncompliant by not taking his medicine at all, taking too much medicine, or not taking it in the amounts and at the times specified.

Reasons for Noncompliance

Some parents don't follow the directions in giving their child his medication because they are having trouble accepting that their child has epilepsy. Sometimes they haven't seen a seizure in quite a while and believe that epilepsy is "over."

Some parents worry about side effects in their children and decide to lower the dose in the hopes of avoiding further side effects. Others increase the dose past the prescribed amount and the blood levels become toxic. Their thinking is that if a little is good, than a lot is better. Parents don't always understand how medications work and it can be harmful to their child to "play doctor."

Occasionally, parents try to scrimp on the dosages to save money. Epilepsy medications can be expensive and some parents figure that missing a dose now and then won't harm their child and will save them money. Other times parents just forget to give a dose and don't bother informing their child's physician. Whatever the reason for not giving the medicine, the result can be the same. The child's blood level can drop and he can have a seizure.

Even if the parents accept the importance of strictly following the doctor's instructions, sometimes their teenager doesn't. Teenagers often rebel against authority with the "You can't make me" attitude.

Teenagers also want to be just like everyone else. They often feel different since they have to take medication. They can feel the peer pressure to drink alcohol or take drugs and know how much more dangerous these activities are for them while they are on antiepileptic drugs.

Another major reason for teenagers not taking their medication is that they feel they have "conquered" epilepsy and it is no longer a problem for them. They may not have had a seizure for quite a while and think they are cured. The other side of this is that they may have poor seizure control even with the medicine and decide that there is no reason to go on with it since it doesn't help. Either can result in serious problems.

Whatever the reason for your teenager not taking his medicine, you must try and make clear to him how vital it is that he take his medication *as directed*. One of the more effective ways to get him to do this is to appeal to him as an adult. Try to avoid treating him as a child. You may need to explain the importance of this issue several times before he is ready to accept it. If it continues to be a matter of control between the two of you, consider having your physician talk with him.

Epilepsy and Developmental Delay

While developmental delays and epilepsy frequently go hand in hand, this is not always the case. The two are, however, often related to the underlying brain disease, which is the cause of the epilepsy. In idiopathic epilepsy, developmental delays are relatively uncommon. Developmental delays are frequently encountered in the symptomatic epilepsies, that are due to an underlying brain disease of either a congenital or acquired nature. When your child is developmentally delayed, he has a fairly widespread neurological impairment.

Occasionally, where your child's epileptic seizure activity is extremely frequent, he may appear delayed in his intellectual development. This happens because of a continued disruption of his brain function by abnormal electrical activity which results in interference with his ability to process information. With the appropriate treatment, this delay can be reversed. Developmental delays are covered in more detail in Chapters 6 and 7.

Prevalence of Epilepsy

Studies show that epilepsy affects approximately .6 to .9 percent of the population. About two million people in the United States have epilepsy. At least 75 percent of the epilepsies begin before the age of eighteen.

Conclusion

Epilepsy can be a very difficult condition for parents to cope with. It is also difficult for physicians. We have to deal with a condition that often is difficult to diagnose in its early stages. And yet we feel the need to diagnose quickly and get your child stabilized as soon as possible. We must then design and implement a program which includes deciding whether to start treatment and what kind of treatment is best.

You, as parents, are entitled to participate in this process and to be a party to information concerning the problem. You should be informed about the diagnosis, including the type of seizure, the elements of the treatment program, the effects of the medications employed and their possible side-effects, and what to watch out for. If the situation is complicated, your physician may want to avail himself of the resources of a neurologist and a comprehensive epilepsy program where the facilities exist for a more precise diagnosis.

Despite the advances in the management of epilepsy in the past ten years, epilepsy is still not fully understood. We still don't have medications which help every child but the outlook is getting better all the time. More children are responding to medications than ever. The development of new drugs is time-consuming and extremely expensive, requiring both animal and human investigation to determine safety and efficacy. Compared to medications for other illnesses, the market for the sale of an antiepileptic drug is not large, and this has further limited the number of antiepileptic drugs which have been developed.

The most promising aspects of future research include prenatal disease detection, the development of vaccines for infectious diseases that have a predilection for the nervous system, and advances in molecular genetics which will allow the detection of biochemical disturbances among those genetically determined epilepsies which we call idiopathic.

Today most children with epilepsy get their seizures under control and go on to live normal, productive lives. They go to college, get married, have children, run in marathons, climb mountains; the list is endless. There is every reason to hope for a brighter future for *your* child, too.

Parent Statements

It does get better. It really does.

One of the most important parts of having a child with seizures is finding a doctor who you can be open with, feel comfortable talking to, who will answer any question—and one who likes your child.

The second after you find out that your baby has infantile spasms, ask for the name of a family that's gone through it. Call them.

When Stephen was fifteen we had a doctor tell us, "I doubt he'll get any better, in fact, I think he'll get worse." I saw the mask fall down over my son's face and I sat and watched him withdraw, literally saw it.

I once heard a woman at a seminar giving a neurologist a pretty hard time about surgery. She wanted her daughter to have it and she said she'd show him articles about it and she'd educate him. He was being very tolerant and finally he looked at her, seemed so exasperated, and he said, "I could take her brain and spread the whole thing out on the table and I still wouldn't be able to see epilepsy."

You learn how long thirty seconds really is when you watch your child having a seizure. Not to mention the eternal amount of time it takes for a ten minute seizure to pass.

I'd have to have been through every drug in the book before I'd put a kid on phenobarb. It really makes them climb the walls. A lot of doctors still give it first and leave them on it while testing other drugs too. What a mix.

The first two months of the ketogenic diet were what we called the dark days. She wouldn't eat. It was a high fat diet; she was in a state of ketosis. No sugars–no carbohydrates. We'd spend an hour or two trying to get her to eat fats, butter, mayonnaise, sausage, whipped cream and then she'd throw it all up. It was very hard on all of us.

It wasn't that we were mistreated in the hospital. We just weren't treated. The nurses attend to IV's and procedures rather than kids with seizures. And we really needed care, believe me.

Your doctor will never see them have a seizure, they always have one as soon as you walk out the door.

We've cut out one drug all together. It was felt the combination of drugs was increasing seizure activity. He's so much more alert, his physical ability is so much improved–he can open a door again.

Our doctor treats a fifteen year old who has Lennox Gastaut who is in high school and will graduate. So the potential is there for our son to do well.

I need to be educated. Don't assume that I know anything. He's my child, I am the parent. I can ask you anything I want to. Just don't keep anything from me. Tell me everything.

It took several months of frustration before they told us how devastating his seizure type would be. We really wish they had been straightforward from the very start.

The doctor told us first we'll have to get these seizures under control then we'll have to look at the long range. This was the first ray of hope we'd seen in six months. He told us he'd seen seizures much worse than this. Then he examined Matthew's eyes and announced he had Batten's disease, a fatal storage disease. As it turned out, Matthew did not have Batten's disease and his seizures were never controlled. The experience with that doctor that day left us feeling defeated and without faith.

I feel very strongly that Matthew's seizures are effected by the humidity and barometric pressure and I wanted them to check that. This one young doctor told me that I'm not capable of recognizing what is a seizure and what isn't a seizure. It has to be a double blind study and it has to be this, and has to be that before it's really that. And I said, "But I really know my own child." When I can sit down and read the weather map and predict whether he's going to have a lot of seizures or not, it bears some discussion.

If I'd give other parents any advice at all, I'd say, "Stick with one drug. Only when you're dead certain that it won't work, consider moving to another drug. I've seen the effects of too many drugs and it is almost worse than seizures."

Doctors do not take into account that we pay them for information so that we can make the decisions as to what is in the best interest of our son. We realize we don't have all their training, but we do want to take part in making decisions.

Until she was six she was very strong-willed and still having tantrums. As soon as she got on that medication, she was a different child. My neurologist does not believe that the medication had anything to do with it.

I'm very concerned about the lack of new medications for people who have uncontrolled seizures. I realize how important it is for the FDA to be thorough in what is approved, but we have not had anything new to try in nine years. That's incredible to me.

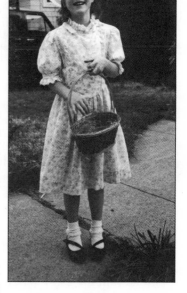

When he has a seizure, if I try to touch him to comfort him, he doesn't respond. He is so alone. I can't get through. I have to stand and just watch him and there is just nothing I can do to make it stop.

I write down the date, time, and what every seizure looks like. Not because I'm really organized, but because when you have to talk to the doctor you're in a mesmerized state of no sleep and no confidence, so if you're writing it down, you can say, on this day and on that day she did this and so.

━━✻━━

We're willing to hear, we're willing to learn, and we're willing to ask questions. I've found that the doctor's basic assumption is that the least amount they can tell you is the most you can bear. It's frustrating.

━━✻━━

When I watch our son having a seizure, I wonder if it is causing brain damage, or if it will somehow affect his intelligence. I know they say seizures don't do those things, but I always wonder anyway.

I think they experiment with drugs—they really don't know what's going to work. Our first neurologist had him on four different drugs and was going to add another. The doctor kept saying seizure disorder, and I wanted him to say yes or no it's epilepsy.

Sometimes it takes the blood lab technicians longer to find a vein than it takes to drive to the lab. We force the technician to stop—we won't let them probe for a vein. And we won't pay, either. Ultimately, it means another trip to another lab, but our son's well-being is our concern.

Sometimes I envy parents who have kids with controlled seizures. We've tried all the drugs, but nothing really seems to work. It's a hit or miss situation and there are no easy answers.

I say, find a doctor you trust, ask a million questions and never hold your tongue.

Our children need their medication to control their seizures, we are forced to accept that. But we must never become overly comfortable with that fact. We must always be on the lookout for developing side effects, level changes, or toxicity to ensure their well-being.

I feel very strongly that parents should follow their own instincts. If they get a doctor who pats them on the head and says "don't worry, they'll outgrow it," I recommend they find someone else.

You know, it's a strange disorder. Some kids who have primary epilepsy do really well and respond to drugs right off the bat. For our child, who has secondary epilepsy, his plight is much more complicated. And his seizures are secondary to a cause that's unknown—no identified cause. It's really a puzzle. I'd rather know the cause. But then there's this hope, too, that science will uncover the mystery.

I can remember him in his infant seat. I took a blanket off him and he gave a little start. I commented, "Well, his moro reflex is intact." Not ever thinking that could be a seizure.

I tell other parents, "You are on your own. Even the best neurologist cannot answer all your questions. You have to go to the library, read a lot, and talk with other parents who have been through it."

Always ask the pharmacist for the insert to the seizure medication printed by the drug manufacturer. Then ask your doctor more questions based on what you read. Always remember, the side effects are potential side effects; they don't usually occur and don't get scared, but be informed.

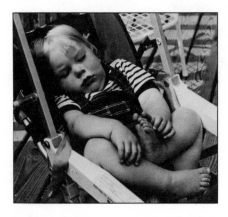

To look at a photo of your child when he was on ACTH therapy is so unbelievable. You just can't believe it's your child. You can't even believe how horrible it was. And then you realize how much of his life you missed. Gone. That whole first year of life gone and the rest is catching up again, you hope.

"I cannot, I will not attempt to tell you what your son's prognosis is, because there is none." Our doctor told us that and I finally just looked at him and understood that it was all a mystery. There was no answer.

I wish he just had tonic/clonic. Everyone can understand them instead of these complex partial seizures where he walks around, snapping his fingers. It looks so odd. Nobody knows what he's doing.

In a sense you need to give the doctors a break a little bit. This is not the chicken pox. They're in a gray area they don't know. Medical science does not know. So how much are you going to get from them, because they just don't know?

It is very important to come to an agreement with your neurologist about what degree of seizure control you both are working toward. Sometimes the doctor will go all out to "fix" the kid. You really must decide if a seizure now and then is worse than lots of medication.

TWO

Your Child's Electroencephalogram (EEG)

DEANNA D. KIRBY, R.EEG-T.*

One of the first tests your child will need to have performed when her doctor suspects epilepsy is the electroencephalogram. This test is absolutely essential and there is no way to avoid it. The probability is that your child will have this test many times in her life and it is a good idea to make it as nonthreatening a procedure for her as possible. It is *not* painful, but can be frightening in that so many unusual things happen to your child all at once. Working together, the technician and you can make the whole experience as pleasant as possible and prevent major problems for the future.

The first time your child has the EEG is crucial to how she views the test in the future. It is sometimes very difficult to get a high quality EEG recording from children. If we can make it easy for her, in familiar surroundings, with people she feels comfortable with, then we can make it an experience that she accepts as part of her life and hopefully, get a more accurate reading. In order to make this a positive experience, you need to know as much as possible about the procedure.

---

* Deanna Kirby is a registered EEG technician and the supervisor of the EEG Evoked Potential Laboratory, Department of Neurology, School of Medicine, University of Virginia.

What Is An Electroencephalogram?

The electroencephalogram (EEG) is a graph recording the electrical activity of the brain. This electrical activity reflects the functional state of the brain at any given moment. Because these electrical impulses are very, very small (they are measured in millionths of a volt) the instrument must amplify them many, many times. The EEG is a tool used in the diagnosis of epilepsy and nonepileptic episodes. When your physician suspects that your child might have epilepsy, the EEG can supply supportive data and provide critical clues as to the type of seizure or seizures your child may have.

The Test Environment

Most children are apprehensive about coming into a hospital. Qualified EEG technicians know this and hopefully will first try to become acquainted with you and your child. Your child's technician should take the time to try to make your child feel comfortable with him and to introduce her to the laboratory in which the testing procedure is to be done. He knows that taking the time now will make the procedure easier for everyone in the long run. If your child knows him, knows the equipment, and the lab, then she will be more relaxed and the test will go much more smoothly. There are many different ways to reassure your child and each technician will have his own favorite techniques. It isn't important how he does it, as long as he takes the time and does it right. The technician welcomes hints on what might work and on helping your child become comfortable with him.

You can help by bringing your child's favorite blanket, a couple of bottles, some toys, and even a cassette recorder with her favorite music. Be sure to let the technician know about your child's moods, her nap time, and anything else you think might be important. Usually I suggest that the parents stay with their child during the test, but if you feel that your anxiety is such that your child could become anxious, then tell your technician and let him decide what is best. You may want to wait in another room.

If you wash your child's head the day of test and don't apply oils or cream lotions, then you will have eliminated one step in the procedure that would otherwise be done at the hospital. This is something you can do at home and will be one less thing for your child to adjust to in the laboratory.

If your child is very young, I prefer to test her after she is fed and around nap time. I prefer natural sleep if it is at all possible. If you can get your child up early on the day of the EEG and keep her awake until her testing begins, then she may fall asleep by herself and everything will be much simpler.

The Procedure

The age of your child and how cooperative she is will determine whether it would be better for her to lie down on a stretcher or to be seated in a comfortable chair. After it has been determined which position is best for her, the technician will measure her head to determine where to put the electrodes.

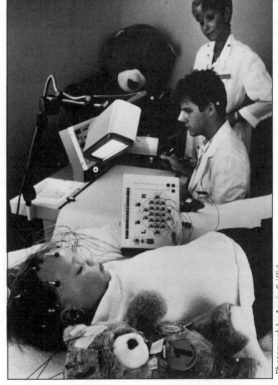

Photograph by Annie Griffiths

When the measuring is done, the technician will then proceed to clean the skin, using alcohol or other solution. Afterwards, he can begin to apply the electrodes. There are two common methods of application, one using electrode cream and the other, most often used for small or restless children, called *collodion application*. Collodion is a liquid that appears like clear liquid plastic sheeting and is applied directly to the electrode or on gauze covering the electrode. It is then dried by using compressed air from an air compressor. There is an odor associated with this method and the hose that carries the air sometimes makes a noise and can be frightening, but is not painful.

At least twenty-one electrodes are applied to your child's head at specific points that have already been measured. Fewer electrodes are used on infants.

I believe in allowing plenty of time for recording. That way the technician can record various stages of wakefulness and sleep. A standard EEG usually lasts between one and two hours. Occasionally a special EEG is performed following sleep deprivation. The child is sometimes wrapped in a sheet or blanket to help her feel cozy. Two activation procedures are used during the EEG. The first is called *photic stimulation*. A light (stroboscopic) is placed in front of your child's eyes, about 25–30cm away. The light is flashed intermittently over a period of time. The second activation procedure is *hyperventilation*. Your child is instructed to breathe deeply or blow a pinwheel for from three to five minutes.

The Results

Technicians know the strain you are under and realize that you want to know the results of the EEG as soon as possible. But we are not qualified to answer all your questions. We are the technical link between your child and your doctor. The EEG is then read by a doctor trained in reading EEGs. The results are then given to your doctor. Your child's doctor has had years of training and is the person best qualified to answer your questions.

Conclusion

All of us, working together, can make the procedure as pleasant as possible for your child. The EEG is a simple, painless procedure and one which your child can come to accept with no fear in the future. By planning the steps in advance, we can all make that first test simple and easy.

Parent Statements

Oh, what can I say about the EEG? Probably the most productive thing I could do would be to get a good primer textbook and learn more about them. I hear there are some doctors who show you different parts of your child's EEG and explain it. Our doctor does not.

It took a whole year to convince our pediatrician and family doctor that something was wrong. Finally they did an EEG and discovered his brain waves were very abnormal.

I went along with Henry for his first EEG. I was really nervous. I still am. I always wonder what his brain is doing in there. What will they find? Will it be worse? What makes it worse?

I would like a tranquilizer for myself on the days he gets an EEG.

Seth vomited after they put the electrodes on for his first EEG. The smell of the cement they used to glue them down made him sick. The woman doing the EEG was trying to be overbearingly friendly with Seth even though it was obvious that he was afraid of her and didn't want her trying to be cozy with him.

I wish the EEG technicians would have everything ready before they put him up on the stretcher. It's only then that they go sharpen their little red pencils, check the paper levels in the machines, get the electrodes unwound, etc.

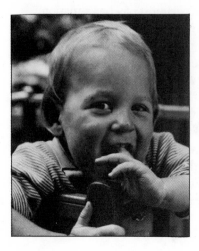

We keep William awake from 5 A.M. until the EEG, which we schedule for the time of day he has the most seizure activity. It is very time consuming and draining on us to keep him awake, but he sleeps during the EEG. Why bother going through all the trouble of an EEG if the kid doesn't sleep?

The technicians that do our son's EEG have tape players and toys. They really know how to help a toddler through this horrible experience. Toddlers have a hard enough time staying in a car seat. Imagine the EEG.

We pretend that our son is going to be a robot and when the technician puts on the electrodes, we turn it into a game.

My husband and I take turns staying with our daughter during the EEG.

I wish I could say something positive about the EEG. For a child what could be worse? For parents, what kind of information does it provide? Usually it's not terrific news!

Our technician has been doing EEGs for fifteen years and does research too. Together we make the most of a bad situation.

It is frustrating not to be told exactly what is on the EEG. Our doctor carefully explained to us that there are many people walking around with epilepsy who have normal EEGs. He told us he'd explain what Matthew's brain waves revealed during the two hours of his life that he was on the EEG – but that it didn't necessarily represent any more than that.

THREE

Adjusting To Your Child's Epilepsy

HELEN REISNER

Right now you are in the midst of one of the busiest, most crisis-filled times of your life. You are suddenly faced with the fact that your child has epilepsy. You are leaving behind your old way of life and are looking at a totally new and bewildering future. You not only have to cope with your own feelings but must also help your family cope with theirs.

Your gradual adjustment to this diagnosis is not easy, but you will get through it. Your family life will one day again be manageable and enjoyable. But in the meantime you will experience feelings that are confusing and, for some of us, overwhelming. This chapter will help you understand your feelings, learn how to work through them, and then turn your attention to helping the rest of your family.

Your Feelings

Epilepsy is one of the most difficult chronic medical conditions parents and children can face. This is because no one can predict when the next seizure will occur—or if it will ever re-occur. There are no answers to questions like, "Will my child's medicine affect his learning and development?" "Will he develop side effects?" "Will he be okay?" "What does his future hold?"

You want all the information you can get and you want a cure. Unfortunately, epilepsy has no cure–only control, and even then only eighty percent of people with epilepsy achieve control. The remaining twenty percent must learn to live with seizures. This reality is very

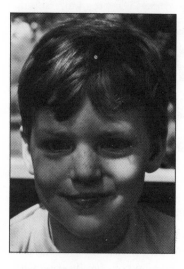

hard to accept. While you are struggling toward acceptance, you may be flooded with feelings that range from anger and rage to denial, pity, and sorrow. Go ahead and feel them.

No matter how "bad" or "shameful" you think your feelings are, they are only feelings. You have the right to any feeling and should not try to pretend it doesn't exist, but rather, experience it, and then work through it. Regardless of how "bad" or "shameful" your feelings are, we have all felt the same way at one time or another. There is no correct order to all the stages of your personal adjustment to your child's epilepsy. Each of us responds individually, and we all go through it.

When you first learned that your child had epilepsy, you were probably stunned. The feeling was overwhelming. You knew something was wrong, but you hoped it was a virus. A fever. Anything. But now you know it's epilepsy. Suddenly your goals and plans are shattered. You simply cannot believe what you've been told. Very few of us knew much about epilepsy when we got the diagnosis and we walked away from the doctor feeling nothing at all. It was like being wrapped in a blanket; we could hear sounds but couldn't identify them. We made it to the car and somehow drove home. We were in shock.

As the shock wears off, your next feeling is probably one of helplessness. You don't know anything about epilepsy and you forgot to ask the doctor so many important questions. The most important one screaming in your head is "What will happen to our child?" You turn to your doctor for guidance, but you feel overwhelmed by his expertise and your total lack of knowledge. You feel intimidated. This is your child, but you are a helpless bystander letting strangers make major decisions. You respond in one of two ways; either you deny the problem or you withdraw. Your feelings are overwhelming and you are no longer in control.

Eventually, as the process goes on, you might begin to feel guilty. "Did I do this? Was it the medicine I took when I was pregnant? Should I have stopped smoking? Is it in my genes? What did I do so wrong that God is punishing my child?"

And then there is the anger. Lots and lots of anger. You blame the doctors, nurses, neighbors, friends, the world for every little thing that happens. You feel so angry at your spouse. "Why can't he/she help? And the other kids are so demanding. Can't they see how worried you are? Can't they help out more? Can't they just be good?" You think the doctors give guarded information and you think there is not another person who understands.

Eventually another powerful feeling emerges—grief. You are so sad now. Your child—the one you knew before his seizures—is gone. You mourn the loss of your healthy child. You want to go to sleep and never wake up. You want your child to just go to sleep and never wake up, or just die painlessly. You could have a funeral and go on with your lives. There is nothing "wrong" with this feeling. It's very common and is just a way we have of trying to avoid the reality of this new burden. The grieving eventually gets done and you can go on with your job of finding the best doctors, the most appropriate drugs, the best possible life style for your family.

One day you wake up, look around, and something is different. You feel better, brighter, and more hopeful. You have adjusted and can look down the new path before you with a fresh feeling. Now you can educate yourself. You can reach out to other parents. You begin to trust yourself and your instincts. Those first feelings of hopelessness, anger, and grief are gone. For now. You have to realize that the feelings come and go with each new crisis, although with time you will be able to face each new crisis without being totally overwhelmed.

You have the emotional time now to take a look around and realize that you have pretty much lost touch with a lot of your old friends. Because they are afraid of your child's epilepsy? Don't be too sure. Maybe they just don't know what to say and aren't sure if you want to hear it anyway. You could have been pushing them away because you were so wrapped up in your feelings.

Some friendships are going to fade away. Perhaps your friends don't understand epilepsy, or are afraid of illness. Whatever. It's not your problem. There will be other friends; both those you already have and those you will make in the future. These new friends are people who can sympathize with what we go through and give us tips on how to go through it more easily. You can find these parents at parents groups. It can make a world of difference to you and how you handle epilepsy.

Helping Your Other Children Adjust

Your other children need to be kept informed on what is going on with their sibling. This child with epilepsy is not just *your* child, he is

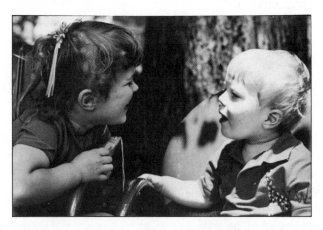

also their brother or sister. Chapter 4 gives you an outline of what to say to your other children, and how to explain epilepsy to them. In this chapter we will concentrate on helping your children adjust to their feelings.

A good rule of thumb is that whatever feelings you have gone through in adjusting to a diagnosis of epilepsy, your children will need to go through, too. They will be afraid that they caused their sibling to get sick. They will be angry at the disruption in their lives. They will dream of death. The difference is that they don't know how normal and acceptable these feelings are. It is your job to make that clear to them.

Get them to express their feelings. Small children can use play therapy to get out emotions. Use a doll, or a TV story, or a book to begin the discussion. "Boy, was Frances angry at her sister. I wonder why? Do you have any idea why Frances was so angry?" After they tell you how they feel, make sure they understand that it is all right to feel that way.

Try to get your children involved in groups that have other disabled kids or siblings of disabled kids. Your children need to know that they are not alone – either in their feelings or in having a special needs brother or sister. Sometimes it may seem that way to them when they look at their friends and everybody else seems like they have a normal, problem-free family life. Getting together with other families with special needs children can reassure them that they aren't "different" from everybody else. In fact, it is one of the most important experiences you can provide for them.

Your Marriage

There's no getting away from it. You are different now. Your spouse is different now. And so is your marriage. Your old life is gone. It seems as if your whole being is tied up in medications, seizures, doctors, and survival. Maybe it is, but it won't always be. When you regain balance and have time to breathe, your marriage will be there and so will your spouse.

You must take the time to learn what your spouse has been going through. You must find out what his/her feelings have been and you must share your feelings. Communicating is the most important step to rebuilding your marriage. You may not know what you want or need from each other any more, but if you can talk about it, then you can both be reassured that you still need each other.

Some parents experience chronic fatigue. Most children have periods where they don't sleep through the night, but children with epilepsy seem to have more interrupted sleep periods than most of us can tolerate. Fatigue has a way of creeping up on us and depleting our strength and ability to cope. Try to work out an arrangement to take turns dealing with your nights so you both aren't totally worn out.

Go out by yourselves one evening a week. To do the grocery shopping in peace, or see a movie, or sit in the library. You may just want to come home and eat dinner quietly before getting hit with all the latest medical news. Talk about your needs and what can be done to get those needs met.

Sharing private experiences together, without children present, is essential in any marriage and hard enough to manage. Now it may seem impossible, but it isn't. Do whatever you have to, but find a reliable babysitter and get out. I don't mean just to parent support meetings. I mean to take a walk in a park holding hands. Or a candlelit dinner. Figure something out on your own. It may not be very frequent, but just the knowledge of an upcoming romantic outing can lift your spirits. One ingenious mother started a babysitting group made up of parents of special needs children. It saved a lot of explanations and worry, and was a marriage saver for a lot of us.

Some of the strongest marriages are those where the partners get support from friends, not just each other. This is usually easier for the wife since she tends to meet more parents in similar circumstances than the husband does. See about finding a men's support group.

In some cases the adjustment to your new life is a little more than you can bear as a couple. Your marriage can begin to feel like a prison with no way out. If you feel this way, it's vital that you make some time for yourselves to be alone and talk or not talk and just have fun.

Make your marriage a top priority. You need each other and your children need both of you. Do whatever you have to. It's not easy, but many parents find that their marriage is stronger, better, and happier than it ever was before.

Your Balancing Act

Don't feel too sorry for yourself. Everyone has to walk a tightrope balancing needs, wants, and demands. Your burdens may seem heavier than most, but since there's not much you can do about it, accept it and plan how to make it as easy as possible. Remember your life has changed since epilepsy; it hasn't ended.

The first thing is not to have tunnel vision. Don't focus on epilepsy to the exclusion of everything else. Epilepsy is just one part of your life. Your other children have needs, your spouse has needs, and your marriage has needs. And so do you! So make a mental plan. Try to chart the necessary items on some sort of daily/weekly schedule and then fit in the rest. If they don't all fit, don't worry about it. They never do. The idea is to at least have a plan to go by.

Try to organize your schedule so that all your children have some time alone with you. Then schedule some time for yourself, your spouse, and your marriage. If you have conquered your weekly schedule so that *most* of what you need to do is included, expand it to a monthly one.

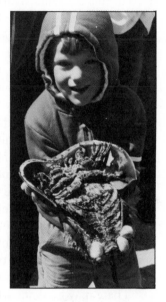

In a monthly planner you can include special family outings. You will have to make some special preparations to allow for your child with epilepsy, but you make special preparations for special circumstances already. Think about it. You never travel without your baby's teddy bear, diapers, and Cheerios. Older children have more sophisticated belongings to bring along like books, tape recorders, and games. Remembering the necessary medical supplies is really no more time-consuming. In fact, keep a special bag already packed near the door or in the trunk of the car with medications and copies of any necessary medical information so you can take off any time. These are added preparations, but nothing to focus on. They're just extras. It's the same with your child with epilepsy.

How about a vacation in this monthly planner? Sure, it's possible. Lots of us go away. It just takes a little extra planning. We carry a supply of medications. We get our doctor to make a referral in case of an emergency. If you don't want to bother getting referrals – don't. Every town has a hospital that's open twenty-four hours a day. There are very few places to go where you can't get to a doctor if you need one. We keep a record with us of our child's condition and find out where the nearest hospital is. If we can't get away for the traditional two weeks, we can usually make a long weekend. You can do it; it just takes planning and a willingness to look for alternatives. When you seriously think about going, there's really no reason not to go.

Becoming Part Of The World Of Epilepsy

That's what this book is all about. We hope to expose you to most of the terms, medications, educational needs, and personal needs you will come up against. But reading this book is only one step. You will need to educate yourself on a continuing basis. Ask questions. Read. There is a detailed reading list at the end of this book that can guide you to other sources of information.

You will also need to develop a family strategy for handling epilepsy. Everyone must be able to deal with a seizure appropriately and explain it to others. Maybe you are great at understanding medical jargon and reading labels but hate taking your child in for tests. Negotiate with your spouse and split the work load. Often your child's therapists and school professionals will accompany you on visits to doctors and hospitals. There is also no reason for both of you to go on every visit, but there may well be a good reason for both of you to go for important consultations. Work out your strategy to include these items.

Who wrestles with the insurance companies? Who handles informing family members of medical changes? What help can you reasonably expect from your other children? You must guard against turning them into little parents, but perhaps they can contribute by doing a few extra chores around the house.

There may be times when your child needs to be hospitalized. Advance planning can lessen the fears all of you may have. Try to take a tour of the hospital in advance. If your children can come too, great! Show them the cafeteria, the waiting room, whatever is appropriate. Then they can visualize where their brother or sister is, and if you're staying there too, then they can picture where Mommy/Daddy is eating. It's something for them to hold on to. Each member of the family should have assigned jobs during the hospitalization to keep things running smoothly. Explain to your other children exactly what will happen to them while you are gone. "Sally, after school you will go straight to Ms. Doe's house until Daddy picks you up."

Epilepsy can be an expensive illness. No matter how good your insurance coverage is, you usually end up spending a lot of money yourself. Plan for it. And in your planning, remember your other children. We found it a good idea to have a small "special" account for each of our other children for those little extras. Instead of always having to say, "We can't afford it," sometimes we are able to say, "Sure, let's take it out of your special account."

Learn the right language to get insurance reimbursements. Your doctor or therapist is a good source of information for insurance claim information. Ask other parents. Try, in all cases, to get a prescription from your doctor for services and items related to services. Don't accept any first refusal to pay a claim. Be prepared to resubmit claims with a letter explaining a medical procedure, the need for it, and why it was done. Keep asking for the next person up the ladder of authority. Becoming a careful consumer can save you a great deal of money.

Conclusion

Stress is a reality when you have a child with epilepsy. In many ways the level of seizure control determines your stress level. No matter what level of control your child achieves, you can learn to handle your own feelings and adjust to your own stress levels. For many, the key is to keep moving. Others need to go slow. Don't get stuck in any of those early feelings we discussed at the beginning of the chapter. Get on with your life. Plan where you can, and accept the fact that there is a great deal of uncertainty with epilepsy. Always climb back up on that tightrope and keep balancing. Remember, epilepsy is only one part of your life; not your whole life or your family's.

Parent Statements

I've got to convince myself that he is not going to die during a seizure. Every time I look at him he's not my son anymore. He's this little thing that's shivering and shaking and his eyes are rolling and he's drooling and he looks like he's going to die. If I can accept that he's not going to die then I think I can accept the whole thing.

Some of our closest, dearest friends are those we've made since Kirsten's epilepsy. It's amazing how automatically close you feel to other people who have kids with epilepsy.

My husband deals with it completely differently. He doesn't seem as emotionally involved. He just deals with it.

Our marriage didn't survive this at all. He's gone. He couldn't handle my response to our child. He's very good with her, but he didn't want to take us both on.

Robbie had infantile spasms at five months. Our pediatrician thought he had an ear infection or some other malady. Does this sound familiar? At nine months it was finally diagnosed. My wife tended to blame herself for taking an occasional cold pill during pregnancy or the DPT shots Robbie got. Finally we got on with living.

Our neurologist told us that our daughter could have a seizure anywhere, anytime. She could have one while swimming, she could have one in class, she could have one while driving a car. She could have one anywhere, anytime. And if my daughter and I worry about it, she'll just have to stay in a little room for the rest of her life.

My so-called "friends" that silently slipped out of the picture are what I now call surface people. Their feelings, compassion, and ability to understand what another person is going through doesn't go very deep. Sometimes you wonder how you could have been friends with them before. Maybe they're afraid. If your child happens to be handicapped or delayed they just don't know how to relate to you.

The only benefit to Bobby's handicap is that his sisters are more sensitive to kids with problems. Any problems. We have a new perspective on life. We don't argue over little things; we understand what is important and what isn't.

I can't believe it when people complain about their kids having a cold or an ear infection. Such trivia in this world. How those people can't cope. They're so helpless and overwhelmed by normal childhood illnesses. I barely have any tolerance left for their complaints.

When we first got the diagnosis I went crazy trying to find the reason. I went back through my pregnancy, my family, my husband's family and then I realized, why does it make any difference? This is what I have.

I felt really lucky that my daughter was normal and devoted all my energy to my son. After about a year I stopped dead in my tracks and realized I was ignoring her.

One of the things I'm finding overwhelming with having a handicapped kid is the extra problems; you have to convince the doctors you know what you're talking about, do piles of paperwork for the insurance company, figure out educational needs, see what legal rights exist. So much extra work on top of the daily care itself.

Some of our friends didn't see us through our rough times. They couldn't accept that we were angry or even in the angry stage. Maybe they don't even know there is an angry stage. I guess we had no common ground. They didn't understand our feeling of loss for our normal child that went away. We lost him to epilepsy.

Seeking a second opinion is such a draining experience on the entire family. We have to go home, regroup, get our nerve back up again and go back out never knowing what's in store for us.

We've become self-educated. No one would offer us any information. We'd observe, we'd read up, and then go meet with the doctor and ask him to verify our observations. We literally self-educated ourselves a step at a time.

Going to the Comprehensive Epilepsy Center really helped us as a family. We learned about drugs and drug levels. This is kind of embarrassing but as parents we thought, this is good, maybe a little more would be better so we sneaked up his meds (without really realizing what we were we doing, we had overdosed him). The center helped us, educated us.

I maintained some old friendships but haven't really discovered how to make new ones. Having a handicapped kid has handicapped me—not her.

I was the one who was in charge in emergencies in the military and now in my business. All of a sudden, after a party where I had had four drinks, my son had his first seizure. This was the night I was called into action! I never, ever drink anymore. Just because we never know what moment we'll need to be prepared. This might be the night I'm called on.

My best friend left his wife in August. He felt life wasn't treating him the way he thought it should. So he left. He changed it. I immediately thought how can he decide he doesn't like his life and change it? I can't change mine, I can't leave. I feel obligated. We have to stay together regardless. Period.

We have been trying to get this under control for years now. We've gone from doctor to doctor. We heard of a new doctor, a new plan, a new hope, but we're now at a point in our daughter's life that we wonder which would be worse—weeks of new tests, drugs, experimenting, crews of young residents and medical students poking around asking the same zillion questions over and over again—or just let her be?

My neighbor told me that she always feels guilty when she comes over to visit with her normal child, because even though she's a year and a half younger, she's still far more advanced. Her daughter's development just zoomed right past my son's.

I am not the supermom of a handicapped kid who's going to be there regimenting his time and pumping him full of all this stimulation. It's more a balancing of both of our needs. My needs have to be met just as much as his in order for there to be a semblance of harmony.

My husband got very depressed. He used to smile a lot; he was assertive; he built a log cabin. He even cut down the trees. Everything! I hadn't realized he was slipping until he hit bottom and all of a sudden there was the wimp sitting there. I thought it must be me, I must be the worst witch in the world. We were in constant crisis. We went to counseling together. He went to a psychiatrist. He was on antidepressants for awhile.

As far as our marriage goes, I'd say he was angry a lot longer than I was. I was the one going to all the meetings and had to cope with it and yet he could just be angry. That was really difficult, going through the acceptance stages.

Even her father had a problem with denial. I was the one home with her, living it. He just went to work. He wasn't there. I was all alone.

I can remember being so angry at my husband because I was doing all this reading. I'd give it to him and say "Read this, why can't you read this? Why aren't you having this compulsive need?" I was so bothered.

I can't stand sitting around listening to people saying how terrible seizures are and acting like it's the worst thing that ever happened. I think it is a matter of acceptance; it's no big deal. You can't do anything to make it disappear, so on with your life.

My friends relate to me differently when they talk about something that's troublesome to them. They always say that it is probably small compared to what we go through. I wish they could understand that their problems are important to me, just like mine are to them. I don't compare who's got it worse.

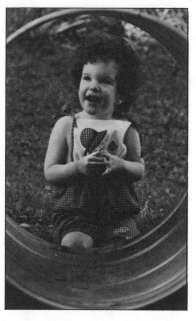

We've missed out on taking family vacations, and doing fun things and worry that we've lost some fun and educational times with Kirsten's sister. We devoted so much of ourselves to Kirsten and to controlling her seizures.

I think withdrawing is a coping mechanism. There's only so much a human spirit can handle.

We're not involved in any extra activities like advocacy or more support groups. We're looking for a little normalcy. What is more helpful – a support meeting or going to the movies?

I have been so tired at times. So depressed. I withdrew. It was a stage. Somehow I have found an inner strength, a sense of courage. A new me has come away from this crisis and I have found that there still can be laughter and joy. We can be happy.

FOUR

Who Do I Tell And How?

HELEN REISNER AND GAIL HENRY*

Both of our children have epilepsy – have seizures – have a seizure disorder.

> *Will began having seizures when he was three months old. He had infantile spasms, which is a very serious type of epilepsy that is often associated with mental retardation and regression and just generally has a grim outlook. He was treated within a month with ACTH, a steroid therapy, and the infantile spasms went away. Some children aren't so fortunate. But he also had, and still has, another type of seizure (complex partial which becomes generalized) that is not controlled. He has a seizure every day, but now that he's on just one drug, he is so much more alert. Sounds odd, but even with his epilepsy and marked developmental delays, he is a joy for us and contributes a lot to our family.*
>
> *Michael had myoclonic seizures. His are completely controlled. Myoclonic seizures are often associated with a more severe underlying condition and mental retardation. When he was diagnosed, we were told two things: "Myoclonic seizures are hard to control. And they get worse." We have been very lucky. There has been no sign of retardation, and the seizures have been controlled*

---

* Gail Henry runs a support group for parents of children with epilepsy and is active in the local EFA affiliate, Epilepsy Foundation/National Capital Area in Washington, D.C.

so well that at age five he has actually begun withdrawal from the drug. We attribute our luck, if you will, to quick action in the early phases and to correct diagnosis and drug therapy. But who knows; it may be just luck. No one really knows for sure why some children respond to the medication and some do not.

The reason we have begun the chapter in this way is to demonstrate how parents might spontaneously talk about their child's epilepsy. One major aspect of having a child with seizures is being a parent of a child with epilepsy. After the diagnosis, the reality of the new situation begins to sink in. Families respond in unpredictable ways. There is no one right way to respond, but there is a right attitude.

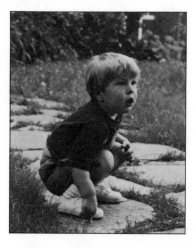

Epilepsy is a condition that requires specialized medical treatment, ongoing attention, and keen observation, as well as social and educational adjustments. We hope to shed some light on how to share the experience of having a child with epilepsy.

Your children are not old enough to truly understand their condition, and they do not have to explain it to their teachers or babysitters. You do. It is those encounters; with yourselves, your family, your friends, your neighbors, your children's teachers, and really the rest of the world that we want you to face with courage and confidence. Never forget that the way you explain epilepsy to others is an example for your child to follow.

First of all, in the opening sentences we used the words "epilepsy," "seizures," and "a seizure disorder." There are many ways to express this neurological condition, this elusive malfunction of the nervous system, this abnormal electrical discharge deep within the brain. People choose to call it different names for many reasons. Some steer away from the word epilepsy because they believe it carries social misconceptions and makes people respond differently than they otherwise would. Others choose to use the term epilepsy because they do not believe it has any undesirable baggage and they have actually formed positive associations with the word and the epilepsy movement. Seizure disorder definitely expresses the idea that the person has seizures and that in some way there is disorder. But the word disorder also has negative implications for some people, so they simply say "has seizures."

As with the group of seizures and syndromes we refer to as epilepsy, the descriptions are as varied and as confusing as the problem itself. There are almost as many names as there are drugs to treat it, and the names are almost as useless as some of the drugs. It would be so much easier if somewhere along the line someone had decided upon precise jargon and everyone around the world had agreed.

In the 1960s the International League Against Epilepsy, through the Commission on Classification and Terminology, did just that: they developed a classification of seizures. As medical research advances and more seizures are identified they are added to the classifications. Now people around the world can, in fact, talk to each other about epilepsy and know exactly what the other person is talking about.

In addition to choosing among general terms like epilepsy, seizure disorder and "has seizures," we must also figure out the differences between grand mal and tonic/clonic, petit mal and absence, psychomotor or temporal lobe and complex partial. It's really no wonder that the public remains uninformed when those of us who are deeply involved are still struggling with terminology. Please refer to the chart on page 238.

Helping Yourself

Before you can tell people about your child's epilepsy, you'll need to get your feelings in order. What do you think about epilepsy? What is the first thing that pops into your mind when you say the word to yourself? Give yourself time to think about this and then sit and talk your thoughts and feelings over with your spouse or best friend. Your goal is to find an easy, comfortable explanation of what kind of seizures your child has and then use it. It is of no help whatsoever to tell another person, "My child has epilepsy." It really doesn't mean much. As one of the people in our parents' support group said, "Better you define it than they do." So it makes sense that the first step is to compose a description, like: "My son has epilepsy. His seizures are called complex partial. If he has a seizure, it's usually in the late afternoon. It begins suddenly, without apparent reason. He stands up and walks backward and forward. He will fiddle with his shirt collar or belt buckle and smack his tongue and lips. Sometimes he talks nonsense. You will not be able to get his attention, because he is not conscious. The seizure usually lasts for about eight minutes and then he sits down, has some jerking movements, and very obviously becomes conscious again. At that point I usually sit beside him, talk softly with him, and generally see if there is anything I can do to give him comfort and support. I explain what happened if he asks and just wait. He is usually worn out and wants to be quiet for awhile."

Information like this is useful, informative, descriptive, non-threatening, and objective. Your child will certainly benefit and you will feel at ease when you leave your child.

How do you get to this point, though? Coming to grips with your child's epilepsy and making this condition just one of the many facets of your child's life is the essential first step. The parents who are able to discuss epilepsy matter-of-factly teach their child that there is nothing odd or embarrassing, fearful or misunderstood about her.

If your child has just been diagnosed, you are still in shock. Hard as it may be to believe, the pain you feel does go away, but not right away. Give yourself time. The feelings of anger, grief, shock, and fear are normal. Every parent we've talked to has experienced precisely the same reactions. Actually, letting other people know that you are angry or fearful about your child's seizures is perfectly okay. You have permission to be sad, to grieve. You have suffered an enormous blow, and you don't need to deny it. If you have to explain to a teacher or babysitter what is going on and you start to cry, so be it. It won't be the first time or the last time that a person has openly wept; it's only human. The person witnessing your emotion has felt similar emotions and will probably appreciate your openness. Eventually you will adjust, and you will be able to explain your child's condition to anyone any time.

Within our parent support group we found that many of us had used similar coping mechanisms during the stages right after our children were diagnosed. We read everything we could get our hands on about our children's particular type of seizure. We haunted medical school libraries. We kept diaries of our children's seizures, medications and possible side effects, blood levels, and visits to the neurologist. It soothed our feelings of helplessness to be doing something, to become better educated. It was therapeutic.

Find a parent support group. There are few experiences that can equal the isolation of having a child with epilepsy, and there is nothing that will shatter the isolation like a few other parents who have been there. It can also be helpful to talk with parents who have children with problems other than epilepsy. You will discover a whole world of families that have special needs children. The strength and inspiration you will gain from them is infinite and the friendships deep and enduring.

If you are at a loss as to how to find a parent support group or someone who specializes in helping people grieving over the loss of a child or adjusting to a devastating diagnosis, call the local affiliate of the Epilepsy Foundation. They are there waiting for your call. They not only have an abundance of pamphlets and printed materials about epilepsy, but are aware of all the local resources and people who can help you. There are also established parent support groups which are led by other parents or professionals. The Resource Guide at the end of this book has other organizations to contact about parent groups.

Most people we know have also had individual or family counseling. This is a crisis and it's best treated like one until you are on solid ground. Most parents have told us that once they finally went to a mental health professional, the relief they experienced was overwhelming. It is vital to be told that your feelings are not only real, but justified. You'd better believe that you've been wounded, need time to heal, and also need some skills for the mending process.

So now let's assume that you have begun to cope with your new child and your new role as a parent. Things aren't going to be like you thought they would, but they're what they are. There is no turning back, so it's time to move on.

Telling Your Child

It cannot be overemphasized that the child herself must be told exactly what she has, why she has it, and what you and she are going to do about it. What you tell your child depends upon her age and emotional state of mind. If you are uncertain about how much information you should provide, STOP. For years researchers have been looking at children's abilities to absorb information. Probably the best advice we can provide is through some examples of stories we've heard from other parents.

One mother told her eight-year-old daughter that when she had a seizure, it was just like a sudden thunder and lightning storm. Every part of the brain rushed to put it out. The brain was so busy working to put out the storm that it couldn't do the rest of the things it usually did, like make her arms and legs work. In fact, the brain got so busy trying to put out the storm, it forgot all about sending messages to the rest of the body, so the body didn't know what to do, and just twitched and jerked around for awhile, until the thunder and lightening storm was out. Then the brain went back to doing its usual job, except it was really tired out from all the work and just wanted to take a nap for awhile.

One mother told her son about the billions of cells in the brain and how there is always electricity running through them, which is how the cells talk to each other. When you want to kick a football, the electricity goes from your brain through the nerves to your foot and causes it to move. Sometimes the brain cells get too active and spread the electricity in many directions. This makes other brain cells pass the electricity on to even more cells. When too many brain cells get excited at once, it is called a seizure. You may pass out, fall down, jerk your arms or legs, or stare into space until the brain is quiet again. Your medicine helps protect these active brain cells like the coating on an electric cord. It keeps the electricity from going in all directions, and that helps keep the brain cells from becoming too active.

The older a child is, the more involved she can become in learning and the more she already knows about herself, her body, and science. Children have natural, built-in, almost instinctive curiosity and appreciate openness.

Build on the natural development of rational and logical thought. Do not overwhelm little children and do not insult older ones. Be sure to include terms the child is likely to hear from others. It is very upsetting for a child to learn that what she's been told is a seizure disorder is really epilepsy. Probably the best rule of thumb is to treat your child as you would like to be treated if you were in her place. Actually, consider the relationship you have with your neurologist. Imagine the perfect relationship – one that satisfies both parties' mutual need for accurate, objective information. What could you do and what could your neurologist do to achieve this relationship? Transpose this line of thought to your child and yourself.

If you are unable to sit and discuss this with your child, find another person to do it. Probably your neurologist is a good starting point. From there you can look to your child's friends or favorite others.

It is very helpful to explain to your child that her epilepsy is invisible until there is a seizure. Explain conditions like asthma, high blood pressure, diabetes. Let your child know that there are millions of people walking around who need medicine to stay healthy. Let her know that if she does not take her medicine, chances are she'll have a seizure. And that the brain does not need to be shocked. It is her job to keep giving the brain medicine to coat the cells to prevent the electrical shocks from getting out of control. That ultimately, it is her brain, her body, her life, and her job to take her medications. Develop a routine with drugs, teach responsibility, and instill self-esteem.

It is also critical to let your child know the cause, if it is known, of her seizures. As with the whole issue, make your approach age appropriate, but be sure to tell her her condition is not her fault. It is not a result of bad behavior. Let her know that she will not die. You may think that you don't have to tell her that, but tell her anyhow. Epilepsy is not terminal.

One little boy, at age three and a half, was having lunch with a few friends at a neighbor's house. After lunch he picked up his medication and dramatically announced, "If I don't take this medicine, I die." His friends gasped in astonishment and admiration, but when his mom heard the story she knew that it was time for another discussion about epilepsy! Who really knows a child's level of understanding? In this case, we find humor in the story, but the child probably wasn't quite sure if he would die or not. The question of death had come up for this child only a few weeks earlier. Although his mother thought she had convinced him that he would not die, he obviously needed more reassurance.

At age five this same little boy was asked about his seizures and why he takes medicine. Without hesitating he responded, "Because I have a bad brain." What he meant or understood about his statement, we do not know; however, we should think about the implications of a small child considering his brain "bad." And it underscores the need to talk with your child frequently to find out how she has internalized all of the information you have given her.

Telling Your Teenager

Teenagers present us with challenges in the shoe store, let alone in the complex world of epilepsy. These are the years of major change, of forceful pulls to independence, to sexuality, to being accepted, ap-

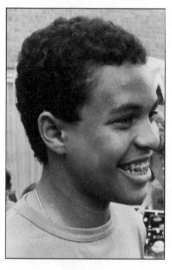

proved of, and to being liked and admired. If seizures complicate and compound the adolescent experience, you can expect a much more difficult time.

It is very hard for teenagers who are in the process of pulling away to turn to their parents for support. But they need it all the same. You will probably have to initiate most of the discussions, and persevere through the common denials of teens. "I don't worry about that." "I'm fine, don't worry about me." "I already knew that; don't bug me." There are lots of them, but the chances are that your child is worrying and doesn't have the answers, so keep opening up chances for you to talk together.

There are several areas of special concern to teenagers that you need to address.

Street Drugs

It may seem a dual message to say "no drugs" to your teenager and at the same time emphasize how important it is that she take her medication. But it's not and you don't need to apologize for your stand. Any caring parent will say "no" to street drugs. Drug abuse is a great destroyer of people and we want our kids safe. Explain that to your teenager and emphasize how much more serious it is for her since she is taking medications that may interact with street drugs.

Friends

If your child is like most teenagers with epilepsy then she is afraid of having a seizure in front of her friends. It is important that you discuss this with her and decide together how to handle it. If she had frequent seizures then the chances of "hiding" them will be small and it's better that she explain to her friends what epilepsy is, what her seizures are, and what they can do to help if she has one when she is with them.

Sex

Your teenager may not express it to you, but she is probably afraid of having a seizure while having sex. We can't recommend how you handle this, there are just too many moral questions involved, but we can tell you that you should know that this is a concern of your child's and you should figure out what you want to say, what you want to recommend, and then open the subject up with your teenager.

Driver's License

This is a very big deal to a teenager. It is her symbol of approaching adulthood and her badge of acceptance with her peers. Whether or not she can get a driver's license will be up to your state regulations and her level of seizure control. Find out and let her know. If she can't drive, try to have some alternative means of transportation to tell her about, but don't expect her to be nonchalant about not being able to drive; it's just too important to her right now.

The Future

There are dozens of questions running around in your child's mind: Will they let me into college? What about getting married? Should I ever have kids? You need to talk about all these questions and more with your child. Don't pretend you have all the answers unless you do. In which case let us know because we'll be facing those same questions soon enough. Be honest with your child; tell her that you understand and sympathize with her fears and that together you will explore solutions. And then do it! Talk with your doctors, read, ask other parents, and ask other teenagers. Together you should be able to come up with some sort of game plan for the future.

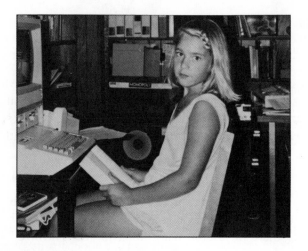

Telling Your Other Children

Secrecy anywhere is harmful. Siblings must be told about epilepsy and what it means for the child who has it. They need to become able to care for their sibling if she has a seizure, and they need to feel free from the responsibility of the care at the same time. The whole issue of siblings is a book unto itself, however, a few thoughts must be kept in mind:

- Children love unconditionally.
- Children strive to please.
- Children imitate behavior.

Many children have special feelings for their siblings with epilepsy, or any special needs. But they also have their own special fears that you need to understand and deal with on their level. At some time any child will feel resentful of all the special attention given the special needs sibling. Children will worry that their brother or sister could die; that somehow they caused epilepsy; that they could get it too; that their parents will blame them for their sibling's latest seizure; and that people will make fun of them, their sibling, and their family. Each age has its special challenges that you will need to face.

You will find that preschoolers are very adept at picking up on your feelings. How you feel about your child with epilepsy will be reflected in your preschooler's attitude. At this age your preschooler won't see a difference on his own so this is a perfect time to teach a positive attitude toward his special needs sibling. You can help foster deep feelings of love and friendship between them that will be the basis of their relationship for the rest of their lives. He will want to help. Let him. Just make sure that he understands that he is helping you do *your job*. This is not his job. He does not need the burden of caring for a special needs child at this age and the feeling of responsibility could carry over to his later years and be a source of great worry for him.

As your child grows a little older (between four and six) he will begin to notice that there is something different about his sibling. Now is the time to use the same basic explanation that we discussed in telling the child with epilepsy only modify it to explain it to your other children. At this age he will probably feel bad about any negative feelings he may have toward his brother/sister and try to hide them. Jealousy is natural between siblings at this age, but your child may try to mask them thinking that it wouldn't be "fair" since his sibling is handicapped. Bring it out into the open and let him express his feelings and get through them. Otherwise he may try to turn into a "perfect" child which will be harmful to him. He is a child, and needs to be free to be one.

By elementary school, your child will need to feel special too. You will have to find the time and methods to bring home to him that he is just as important to you as your child with epilepsy. Show him that although you must spend a great deal of time caring for your special needs child, *his* needs are important too and you make every effort to meet those needs. There will be times when he feels as if his sibling is a giant-sized pain in the neck. One way to defuse those feelings and not have him feel guilty about them is to acknowledge them. "Yes, I know how hard it is not be able to go to the beach this year because Dana needs to be home for special testing. I certainly understand how angry you must be at all those tests Dana is having." Turn the feelings toward the event and away from the sibling. It is much harder to stay angry when someone understands and sympathizes with you and much healthier to get angry at an event (tests) than a person you care for. Particularly when you know it really isn't her fault.

As your child reaches adolescence, he becomes more self-absorbed and has less time to devote to his sibling. He will want to be

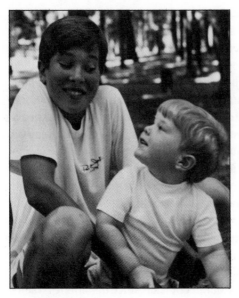

free of the responsibility of caring for his sibling and will resent too many demands on his time. Try to keep from making him into a teenaged parent substitute. Start discussing your plans for the future so that he knows that your child is not his lifelong responsibility. Talk to him about his feelings about his siblings. Don't judge them. Try to keep the golden rule of therapy in mind. "Feelings are neither good nor bad; they just are." Sympathize with any feelings of embarrassment he may have. At this age everything embarrasses them from having the wrong color car, to the wrong color shirt. Try to see how hard having a different brother or sister may seem to him. Let him know that these feelings will change as he grows older. He probably feels terrible that he is embarrassed and wishes he were stronger. If you have to, make deals so that he can have his own space and yet not totally deny his sibling. In one case, a parent negotiated certain events where the sibling with epilepsy didn't come. The teenager was afraid that his sister would drool and have a seizure right in the middle of his football game. So his sister didn't come to the football games. In exchange, the teenager continued to go out for Sunday pizza with the family, even though he was sure to run into some of his friends there.

Telling Other Family Members

Telling the grandparents might be one of the hurdles you will find more difficult. Our parents were raised in the days when children with handicaps were not a part of the mainstream. Retarded children were often institutionalized. Children with epilepsy were often hidden because, until recently, there were no drugs to control seizures. Institutions that accepted retarded children were not always capable of caring for children with uncontrolled seizures. Our parents are products of an era that no longer exists for children with epilepsy. We are entering a new world of thought. Science is revealing the condition for what it is, and parents of children with epilepsy are making sure the word gets out. Therefore, when you tell your parents, you potentially face the need to explain a lot more than you will for your child's teacher. Telling parents is even harder because they are so special, and it may be quite painful to inform them that their grandchild has something wrong with her. Be prepared to accept the fact that they, too, may go through all the same stages of denial and slow acceptance that you yourself did. You will also have to recognize and deal appropriately with the reality that grandparents tend to be very overprotective. If your parents are responsible for the care of your child, be sure to stress that your child must be treated normally and not denied normal rambunctious play. Most of us have found our parents to be a tremendous source of support.

And Then The Rest Of The World

After your family and friends have been brought into the fold and hopefully feel comfortable with your child's seizures, there will always be just one more person to tell. The list goes on and on. It is not necessary to name each person or group of people that have to be told. However, there are babysitters, educational professionals, and other health care providers whom we'll discuss in detail below.

The question of whether to tell anyone or not greatly depends on whether your child's seizures are controlled. Ultimately, it is your decision. If, however, you do not tell people, at some point you must reconcile your fears with your child. You will be sending a dangerous message to your child: epilepsy is something to hide. Please don't do that. It is how you portray epilepsy that determines how others react. Most people initially act like they're not sure what to say or if they should say anything at all. But once they realize that you are very comfortable talking about it, they have a lot of questions and are anxious to gain a better understanding of epilepsy.

Another consideration is your child's safety. Every person you talk to about epilepsy is one less person who might one day force an object into your child's mouth to keep her from swallowing her tongue or who might walk by your adult child as she seizes on the sidewalk because they don't know how to help and are afraid. Most of the parents in our support group have found that people are grateful for information on how to handle a seizure, no matter how unlikely it is.

Basic Information For People To Know About Your Child's Epilepsy

1. The type of seizure your child has and exactly what happens.
2. How often your child has a seizure and at what time of day.
3. The last time your child had a seizure.
4. The kind of medication and dose your child is on, when she takes it, and how it is taken (pill, liquid).
5. What kind of first aid and emergency care is required, if any. For example, for tonic/clonic seizures, try to loosen tight clothing, roll on side if possible, move hard objects, and stand by. For complex partial, stay nearby, keep person from hurting himself by walking or bumping into hard objects, try to coax him into sitting down when it's over.
6. What state your child will be in after a seizure and what kind of care should be provided afterward.
7. Whether or not you want to be called immediately.
8. That you would like to know if there was any behavior prior to the seizure that an observer can recall. This will help you and your child determine if an aura is present and will help with future seizure "breakthroughs." If the teacher or child is aware of a seizure coming on, safety precautions can be taken.
9. That it is impossible to swallow the tongue. **DO NOT** put anything in the mouth.
10. Seizures are not painful.

The School

Make a special appointment each school year to sit down and talk with the school nurse, the teacher, the guidance counselor, the principal, and any sports coaches and extra-curricular activities supervisors. It is absolutely critical that they begin to learn, accept, and take part in the epilepsy movement as informed advocates. One hundred thousand people are diagnosed each year, and seventy-five percent of all epilepsies are diagnosed before age eighteen. Since our children spend a large portion of their time in the education system, it only seems logical that school personnel should become better educated about epilepsy. They must also help us in our advocacy efforts to diminish old stereotypes and to dispel myths. It becomes our role to assist them by being open, frank, matter-of-fact, and comfortable. If you sense any negative reactions, simply express your thoughts about those negative feelings. You can tell the other person that you understand his reaction, in fact might have felt that way yourself, but have since become informed and it is your mission to help him as well. The teacher especially can make presentations about seizures in class. There are teenagers with epilepsy who belong to teen support groups and can come and speak to classes. The local affiliates of the Epilepsy Foundation have speakers' bureaus and an excellent School Alert program that provides a variety of educational materials.

Swimming And Epilepsy

One of the parents interviewed for this book has a teenage son who has been swimming since he was a young child, and has continued to participate on the swim team competitively since his diagnosis. In fact, one of the first seizures that was ever recognized by anyone was seen by the coach. He stated that as Stephen was swimming laps, he just stopped for a few seconds. His right arm went up and he didn't move, then he went on swimming. Since that time, Stephen has developed complex partial seizures and has been through most of the antiepileptic drugs and surgery to try to control his seizures. All without success. However, Stephen has remained on the team and swims each day.

There are some special precautions that must be taken for swimmers. A person with epilepsy should not swim alone. The people with whom he swims should be aware of his condition and possible first aid measures. If swimming when a seizures occurs, the person's head should be supported and tilted to the side. After he is taken out of the water, check for breathing and perform artificial respiration if necessary. Emergency care and a careful medical exam is necessary to check for ingestion of water. In Stephen's case, this kind of care was not necessary because his seizures were not convulsive. If, however, a person has a seizure, it is best to err on the side of caution.

Babysitters

You must go out without your children every once in awhile. In order to enjoy your time away, you need to find competent babysitters. In your initial contact with a babysitter, you inform him of the fact that your child has seizures. Even if your child's seizures are completely controlled, think about the ramifications of a seizure breakthrough. What if the unpredictable epilepsy acts up when you are not there, and you have given no forewarning to the babysitter? It's not fair to anyone concerned.

The collective experience from our support group is that most young people are open and willing to learn about seizures. Again, the bottom line is that most people want to know about epilepsy, want to learn what care is needed, and will usually reflect the same open attitude that you present. One mom in our group simply states that if she ever runs into someone who seems unsure, she doesn't want him providing care for her children anyway; she doesn't hire him.

If your child has uncontrolled seizures and you are looking for a specially trained person, there are many sources to consider. The special education departments at local colleges and universities are an excellent resource. Students studying special education are already committed to caring for kids with handicaps. Nursing schools offer a rich source as do day care centers or high schools where teens are studying child development. Special interest groups, like the Association for Retarded Citizens, often have lists of trained sitters. The Resource List at the back of this book is a starting point. If the agency you call can't help, the person usually can refer you somewhere else. Probably the very best resource is another parent. Call the affiliate of one of the national organizations for leads on parents who live nearby.

Once you have your sitter and you are ready to go out, what preparation and information should you provide? The following brochure has been reprinted with permission from the Comprehensive Epilepsy Program, University of Virginia. It was created by Ramonda Haycocks, RN, MSN. It is also an excellent resource for teachers, camp directors, and anyone else who might care for your child.

SEIZURE INFORMATION FOR BABYSITTERS

Babysitting for any child is a big responsibility. Babysitting for a child who has a seizure disorder may also mean meeting special needs of the child. The information in this pamphlet is intended to help you learn more about seizures, and some helpful things you can do to meet the special needs of a person who is having a seizure. Hopefully this information will make you more comfortable while caring for a child with a seizure disorder. The most important thing to remember is that between seizures the child is just like every other normal, active child. Always treat the child the same as you would anyone else in your care. A seizure is like an electrical storm in the brain. A generalized tonic-clonic, also call grand mal, seizure where a person loses consciousness, falls, becomes rigid and then experiences jerking movements of the body can be a frightening event for anyone who has never seen one before. A tonic-clonic seizure, however, is only one kind of seizure. Other kinds involve unconscious staring spells, or jerking of only certain body parts.

STOP - Before you read the information inside this pamphlet, make sure the child's parents leave the following telephone numbers for you in case a seizure occurs while you are in charge:

FIRST AID _____
TO REACH PARENTS_____
NEIGHBOR_____
PHYSICIAN_____

Keep this pamphlet, or another list of these numbers, next to the telephone so you can always find them. A seizure does not cause any pain, and it is not likely to damage the brain. Sometimes a person is injured from falling as he loses consciousness. Sometimes the person makes an abnormal sounding shrill cry at the beginning of a seizure, or has "funny feelings" and knows that a seizure is about to begin.

WHAT TO DO: If you see the beginning of a seizure try to prevent a dangerous fall by moving the child to the floor. Remove any hard or dangerous objects that the child might bump into and injure himself more. If possible, put a cushion, rolled up towel, or something else soft under the head. Do not try to hold the child still or stop the movements. It is impossible to stop or shorten a seizure—it must run its course. It is common for a person having a seizure to drool or froth at the mouth. Biting the tongue also happens and may make the froth slightly bloody.

WHAT TO DO: Turn the child on his side so he will not choke on the saliva, and continue to hold him on his side until the seizure is over. Do not force a hard object between clenched teeth; the child is in no danger of swallowing his tongue, and you risk breaking his teeth or getting bitten. A person having a seizure may hold his breath for what seems like a very long time—so long in fact that he turns bluish in color.

WHAT TO DO: Stay with the child and watch the seizure. Breath-holding, especially until the child turns blue, is frightening but almost never causes any damage and the child will start breathing again by himself. You can loosen tight clothing, such as collars and waists, to help ease breathing. Sometimes a person will vomit just before a seizure, or wet or soil himself during the seizure. This causes a lot of embarrassment.

WHAT TO DO: When the seizure is over help the child clean up in a calm, matter-of-fact way. Try to reassure the child and make him comfortable to reduce embarrassment. The jerking movement part of the seizure should not last more than 10 minutes. However, it sometimes takes much longer, even hours, for the child to become fully conscious and awake. During this recovery time the child may act confused, "spaced out", irritable, drowsy, or sleepy. The child may also complain of sore muscles.

WHAT TO DO: Stay with the child and make him as comfortable as possible. Allow him to sleep if he wants to. You can gently rouse the child now and again to check consciousness.

GENERAL POINTS:

Always stay with the child until the seizure is over, and observe how it affects the body parts.

Look at a watch or clock if possible so you can get some idea of how long the seizure lasted.

If the child has staring spells, talk to him and ask him questions so you can tell when consciousness returns.

When the seizure is over, telephone the child's parents and tell them of the seizure.

VERY IMPORTANT: If the jerking movement part of the seizure lasts more than 5 minutes, or if there is one seizure after another in a 5 minute period, you should leave the child and phone for FIRST AID. Phone the parents after you call for first aid. Then return to the child and stay with him until help arrives.

QUICK SUMMARY OF WHAT TO DO:

Move child to floor and make environment safe.

Turn on side to prevent choking.

Do not force hard objects between teeth.

Loosen tight clothing.

Stay with the child until seizure is over.

Make child comfortable after seizure.

Call first aid if jerking movements last longer than 5 minutes, or if seizures occur one after another in a 10 minute period.

Phone parents.

SPECIFIC INFORMATION ABOUT _____
                                (child's   name)
Usual kinds of seizure _____
_____

Usual behavior during a seizure _____
_____
_____

How often do seizures occur? _____

_____

Under what conditions is one likely to occur?_____

_____

_____

_____

Medications: list names, dosages, times,and who gives
them _____

_____

_____

_____

Additional information and/or instructions _____

_____

_____

_____

Comprehensive Epilepsy Program
University of Virginia
RJH/1985

Health Care Providers

Let other health care providers know about your child's epilepsy.
One family's dentist was not told about a patient's epilepsy. The patient
seized shortly after the dentist had administered anesthesia. Needless
to say, the dentist didn't know if the seizure was a reaction to the anes-
thetic or was a pre-existing condition. She had no idea what medications the patient was taking, and if there could have been a reaction to
the combination of drugs and anesthesia.

Even a physician recommending an over-the-counter medication
like cough syrup needs to know about your child's antiepileptic
medications. Lots of drugs don't mix. It never hurts to double-check

with a pharmacist before administering any other medication, prescribed or over-the-counter.

Who Else Needs To Know?

It is up to you. You are the best judge. Your child is a good resource as far as helping you decide. You should keep in mind that it is to your child's advantage to have informed friends, teachers, and camp counselors who know proper first aid. And more importantly, these people will have had a chance to think about epilepsy so that they will react in the way you want them to. Your child's friends will take their cues from how grown-ups handle seizures. An informed adult becomes an advocate for your child and for all children with epilepsy.

Beyond the medical implications the dilemma, "Who Do I Tell and How?" is the single most contemplated issue among families living with epilepsy. It is always a point of discussion and concern. Should we tell? Why should we tell? What will happen if we don't? Why does it matter? What will other people think? How will they react? We experience worry, frustration, and uncertainty. All these concerns are normal, valid, and are experienced by all of us. But we cannot get stuck in those feelings. We must reach out, take risks, and be brave. Your confidence will be bolstered with each new encounter and your courage will grow every time you discuss your child's epilepsy. You will be helping to create a new world of understanding so that your child can grow and thrive and look forward to a future free of misunderstanding. The crux of the issue is simply, HOW you tell. There are no guarantees that you will never have to face rejection. To deny the uninformed reactions of others is probably as useless as living in fear of them. You must matter-of-factly accept that epilepsy does present social hurdles that some other conditions do not, but those hurdles will continue to exist only if we do not become advocates for our children and for epilepsy.

If we want the world to view our children as they really are, vital, loving kids who happen to have epilepsy, then we must keep epilepsy in the proper perspective. Our casual acceptance will become the world's. And that accepting world is where we want our children to grow and thrive.

Parent Statements

Sometimes I'll say seizures, sometimes I'll say epilepsy. It all depends on who I'm talking to, what mood I'm in, what we're talking about and if I want to expend the energy.

In the grocery store she began unpacking the cart behind us, looking for the plastics. She likes the feel of plastic. I just turned around and said to the person behind me, "I'm sorry, she's handicapped and likes plastics. If you move your cart a little, she won't bother you. " Then I went home and cried.

I've found that other people really want to ask questions but don't. I've found so many people out there with handicapped kids, or special needs kids, or kids with a problem, whatever you want to call it. And I've found so many compassionate and understanding people.

The status of our mind set as far as Richard's control goes is that he's in pretty good control. We never really know though if he's going to have a seizure. He could. So we do try to let people know if he's going to be away from us. It's a real dilemma. We can't not tell people, because there is this very remote possibility that he'll have a seizure. And then why should we tell them, because he hasn't had a seizure for so long.

His first seizure was during gym class in school. That was five years ago and we just assume that it's on his records now. We never talk to his teachers about side effects or anything. We just hope that we don't ever have to either.

I have a hard time telling people about his epilepsy. I have had a very hard time with it the whole way.

I see all these other sixteen-year-old kids driving their cars and doing this and doing that. That was very hard for Stephen last year. And of course, he has a younger sister who will drive and is going to do all the things he should have been able to do.

We tell people so they don't feel odd about asking, and if we help educate one person, it may make it easier for others. After all, if someone really doesn't want to know, they can change the subject.

You are your child's best and at times, only advocate. You must be very informed and on the pulse of the situation. For example, more than once the pediatrician would have prescribed an antihistamine for a cold if I hadn't reminded him it wouldn't mix with his antiepileptic drug.

Our support group has parents of children with a variety of handicaps—from behavioral problems to physical ones. We have a topic or just discuss our experiences like, "What do you say to the cashiers in the grocery store when they ask probing questions about your kid?" We talk about how it feels to develop new lifestyles, not to get invited to the neighbors, to have to explain, explain, explain all the time.

It always amazed me how everybody appeared to be healthy before my son got sick. Then during casual conversation with neighbors and friends, it seems that seizure disorders come out of the closet.

— �֍ —

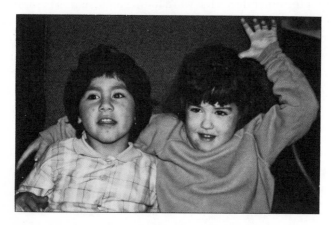

We do not tell a lot of people. It's not a secret; if it comes up in conversation, I won't change the conversation or avoid it. I just feel that it's important for Richard to live free of the consequences of people knowing.

— ✷ —

Apparently a lot of parents feel they have to protect their children. From what? Seizing in public? You can't stop it.

— ✷ —

One time I hired a babysitter and just forgot to tell her beforehand that my son has epilepsy. When she got there, I told her and her face just dropped. It was a look of fear, panic, totally foreign information, a "What am I supposed to do now" expression? I really laid it out to her that this was no big deal, he's not going to die, to swallow his tongue, hurt himself, he's just going to get fussy after it's over and almost begged her to stay.

I am just beginning to use the word epilepsy. I actually used it in a letter the other day. That word for me represents a memory of a girl who came to our high school. She was pretty, she was really smart, all the boys were crazy about her. I just thought she was wonderful. But everybody whispered, she had this terrible thing. She had seizures occasionally. She wasn't under complete control. She was only in our school for one year and she did seize. Oh I don't know. I just remember how everyone whispered.

After soccer season last year, I told the coach that Richard had a seizure disorder. The coach looked at me with such a flabbergasted expression and said "Why didn't you tell me?" And I said "Because you would have treated him differently than you did. Instead, he was treated just like everybody else out there and expected to do everything everybody else did. "

We were advocates for adequate training of school bus drivers. We wanted to make sure that they knew the difference between "a little seizure" and a chain-seizure (status) that required immediate life-saving medical intervention.

I wrote to the National Information Center for Handicapped Children and Youth and asked for their Parent Contact List in my state. I found it a great source.

I like to think that how people react is their problem. That may sound naive, but in anyone's life, being overly concerned with the opinion of others can be very destructive.

FIVE

Helping Your Child Develop High Self-Esteem

WILLIAM R. STIXRUD, PH.D.*

PART I: YOUR CHILD'S SELF-ESTEEM

You may wonder why a separate chapter in this book is devoted to the topic of self-esteem. The reason is simple: helping children develop high self-esteem is one of the most important things that we can accomplish as parents. Knowing this can help to clarify our thinking about what we are trying to do as parents and help focus our goals for our children.

Clarification of our role as parents is much needed these days. Most parents would agree that raising children in the 1980s is very challenging and often confusing. There are few agreed-upon standards regarding what children are supposed to be like and even less agreement about how to discipline and raise them. The extremely fast pace of life, the high rate of divorce, the large percentage of mothers who work full time, the fact that children today know that they have certain rights and are willing to challenge their parents on them – all these factors make parenting a very challenging task, even for parents of

---

* William Stixrud is a neuropsychologist in private practice in the District of Columbia and is also director of the Washington Parenting Center.

youngsters without physical or mental difficulties. Parents in vast numbers need help in figuring out what they are "supposed to be doing" as parents.

Parents of a child with epilepsy must deal with additional challenges and face an even stronger need to become "expert" parents. Notice I said "expert," not "perfect." What this chapter offers is a guiding principle for parents of children with epilepsy – the importance of high self-esteem in their children along with suggestions for accomplishing this most important goal.

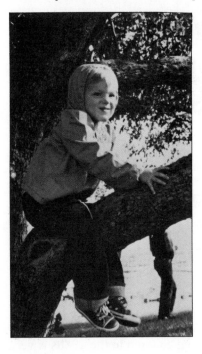

Why is Promotion of Self-Esteem So Important?

Almost everyone writing in the fields of education, motivation, human potential, achievement, success, and personal development is saying that high self-esteem is the single most important asset a person can "possess." High self-esteem allows a person to set high goals, to take the risks which are necessary for success and achievement, and to persist in striving toward goals, even in the face of setbacks. High self-esteem provides the basis for enjoying ourselves and others and for satisfaction with our lives. High self-esteem also provides a sure basis for mature relationships with others.

Certain expressions of the fundamental importance of self-esteem have almost become cliches ("If you can't stand to be alone with you, how could anyone else?" "You can't really love others unless you love yourself"). Yet they are true. It truly is impossible to like or enjoy life without liking or enjoying ourselves, and it is impossible to give others what we do not have. We can need others and be grateful to them for meeting our needs, but we cannot genuinely love them without self-love. In my clinical work with adults, virtually all therapy is self-esteem therapy, focused on healing the individual's relationship with his own self as the basis for improving all other relationships. It is always the case that when a person develops higher genuine self-esteem, relationships with others become more harmonious and loving, and a person becomes more able to pursue the things in life which he desires.

In addition to this "philosophical" justification of the importance of self-esteem, there is ample research evidence to support the idea that the major goal of parenting should be to nurture self-esteem in children. Studies of successful adults have revealed that self-esteem correlates very highly with achievement, while low self-esteem is associated with substance abuse, learning problems, truancy, destructive behavior, and suicide. People across the country are responding to what some writers have called an "epidemic of low self-esteem" by introducing self-esteem into the curriculum of school programs for children and adolescents. The state of California even allocated $750,000 for the study of ways to improve self-esteem in young people as a way of decreasing crime.

Many parents are surprised to learn that self-esteem has more to do with success than do other factors usually believed to be extremely important for success in adult life. Perhaps most surprising is the finding that virtually no correlation exists between grades earned in high school or college and success in later life. Research and clinical experience have shown that high self-esteem is far more useful to a child than 15 IQ points or an extra grade level in reading.

What Is Self-Esteem?

Self-esteem is the way you feel about yourself – your overall judgment of yourself. It involves your own evaluation of your self-worth and your levels of self-acceptance, self-liking, and self-approval. High self-esteem implies a quiet feeling of comfort with one's own being. High self-esteem is not to be confused with a sense of superiority, a need to brag, or a tendency to act better than others – all these reflect attempts to compensate for low self-esteem and feelings of not being good or important enough. Self-esteem is not related to family wealth, level of education, or IQ.

High self-esteem in children is shown in several ways. These include a strong interest in developing skills and abilities, genuine interest in and concern for others, ability to think independently and make independent choices, and confidence in one's own self-worth. Children with high esteem also typically display several of the following characteristics: they feel liked, wanted, and accepted; they enjoy life with enthusiasm; they assume a high level of responsibility for their own lives; they have a high level of self-direction and do not need continual praise and reassurance; they express feelings easily and can admit mistakes without feeling ashamed or excessively guilty; they can be alone without feeling lonely; they approach life with trust and optimism. The self-confidence and self-respect associated with high self-esteem make children able to say "no" to drugs, alcohol, and other dangerous temptations.

Can A Child With Epilepsy Enjoy High Self-Esteem?

Children with epilepsy face many difficult challenges to feeling good about and accepting themselves. For example, the loss of control associated with seizures in itself undermines a child's sense of competence, which is an extremely important aspect of self-esteem. The limiting of athletic and recreational activities which is sometimes necessary can further jeopardize the child's sense of competence and his conviction of being generally "good enough." Children with uncontrolled seizures also have to live with the possibility that they will embarrass themselves in school and have to deal with the very real possibility of teasing and social rejection. In addition, the high level of worry and anxiety which often "surrounds" epilepsy can heighten a child's own natural concern about his health and safety and fuel "irrational" worries, e.g., that seizures are contagious.

Experiences within the family also contribute to the difficulty some children with epilepsy have in developing a strong sense of self-worth. Children with epilepsy are more likely to get the message at home that they are not as smart as their siblings or that they cause more family problems than their brothers and sisters. If parents frequently demonstrate feelings of anger, shame, or guilt regarding their child, these messages can convey to the child that he is not accepted and respected as he is, which makes it difficult for the child to accept and respect himself. When a child or teenager does not accept and respect himself, it is not uncommon to see exaggeration of the limitations actually posed by epilepsy or a tendency to deny the reality of epilepsy, both of which are detrimental to self-esteem. For instance, a teenager may tell his friends he didn't try for a scholarship because his medications won't let him study hard enough to keep up academically, when really he is afraid he is just not smart enough.

Yet despite the daily challenges to self-esteem, achieving high levels of self-acceptance and self-liking is entirely possible for children with epilepsy. In my clinical practice, I encounter many children who are at risk for low self-esteem. Children with learning disabilities, physical handicaps, epilepsy, disabling head injuries, alcoholic parents, and other family-disrupting problems all suffer more assaults on self-esteem than children without these problems. However, while there is a risk of self-esteem problems, there is no reason why children with any impairment or combination of impairments cannot experience high self-esteem. I frequently encounter severely disabled children from very low income families who have far higher levels of self-liking and self-approval than children with lesser problems and greater advantages.

For parents of children with epilepsy there are often so many day-to-day things that must be attended to that focusing on self-esteem may seem like a luxury. Indeed, these parents face an enormous range of problems which consume time, money, and emotional energy. These problems are related to the severity and degree of seizure control, the presence of accompanying physical, mental, or emotional handicaps, and the financial status of the family. Challenges can range from helping an otherwise perfectly normal child with well-controlled seizures live a normal life to helping a multi-handicapped child with uncontrolled seizures who needs constant special attention and protection, and about whom life-and-death concerns are very real.

Despite these problems and concerns, high self-esteem is still the cornerstone for success and happiness and is one of our highest priorities as parents. There are many people with every conceivable gift of nature who harbor strong feelings of self-doubt and unhappiness, and there are others whom nature has appeared to saddle with extraordinary burdens who shine forth in splendid brilliance. It is possible, no matter how severe a child's seizures or how extensive the related problems, to focus on nurturing high self-esteem.

Fostering Self-Esteem In Children With Epilepsy

Unconditional Love

For children to develop the conviction that they are lovable and worthy of happiness, they require a healthy daily dose of unconditional love from their parents. Unconditional love is love without demands. Loving children unconditionally means to love them as they are, no matter what they say, feel, think, or do. This unconditional love is the basis of our relationship with our children.

Being loved unconditionally is not the only ingredient necessary for high self-esteem, but it is an essential one. Children who feel continually pressured to be different than they are develop the idea that they are not and can never be good enough. Children do not do well when they feel that they have to earn their parents' love or when they feel that their goodness as a person in their parents' eyes depends on their behavior or performance. In my clinical experience with disabled children, the extent to which the parents can lovingly accept the child as he is is reflected by the happiness and adjustment of the child.

Challenges to Loving

Many of the parents I work with report that it is extremely difficult to love their child with epilepsy unconditionally. There is often a strong tendency to wish the child were different and to compare the present condition with what "might have been" or what was "supposed to have been." Parents sometimes get "stuck" in an early stage of dealing with having a child with epilepsy and have trouble fully accepting the child as he is.

Parents who work through these feelings of anger or denial often find that they can accept their child's life as it is, while at the same time wanting the best possible future for him. It sometimes helps to recognize that no human being knows what a child or a child's life was *supposed* to be like. This recognition can help you lessen the tendency to sadly compare what is with what might have been. It is also *crucially* important for you to know that even though your child has epilepsy, it is okay for you to love the child one hundred percent as he is, no matter what the reaction of others may be.

Some parents—particularly those whose children's behavior is extremely difficult to manage—report that they no longer feel that they love their child. Such a recognition is, of course, extremely painful for a parent who wants to love his child. It is, however, a necessary recognition and the first step to re-establishing the loving connection that once existed. Professional counseling is often necessary to facilitate this process. For most parents, however, following the suggestions below will help them ensure that their child feels genuinely loved, prized, and enjoyed.

Focused Attention

Communicating unconditional love is not easy, although we generally take it for granted that children actually *feel* loved. In my clinical experience this is often not the case, as children are frequently confused about their parents' feelings toward them. They ask, "If they love me, why do they yell at me all the time?" or, "If they love me, why do they criticize me?"

There are several ways to convey unconditional love to a child that will help the message get through. The most important is what is called "focused attention" or "genuine encounter." This means simply "being here now" with a child, which for busy or pressured parents is no easy task. Focused attention means being alone with your child and giving him your undivided attention without the newspaper or television on. Focused attention can be given in times of your child's need of special attention, but can also be given on a regular basis through spending time alone together. During this "private time" you do not need to teach, scold, or "improve" your child in any way. The focus is just on being together and enjoying each other. A child who feels genuinely enjoyed comes to feel that he is genuinely enjoyable and capable of producing happiness in others.

When giving your child focused attention, the activity of being together *is* the agenda. It is a time when other things are put aside. Doing something with all the children in the family together does not do the trick. A parent needs a private and personal relationship with each child and it is necessary for the child to feel that he is special. It would be very difficult to develop a close relationship with an adult without some "private time" for talking and getting to know each other, and the same is true for relationships with children. As children get older, they require somewhat longer blocks of time in order to open up and communicate with their parents.

Having this private time on a regular basis is extremely important. Because of its powerful effects on children, it is the first thing I recommend to families. The nonverbal message a child receives through focused attention is that he is important enough for his parent to put everything else aside and just be with him. For that time the child feels like the most important person in the world. Many children love to have their private time with parents recorded on a calendar or in the parent's daytimer; in this way they see that it is a special priority for the parent.

This conscious decision to give your child focused attention on a regular basis can be made at any time, although it is easier to decide than to do. The amount of time that most parents spend alone with their children is extremely small, and I have worked with children who cannot remember the last time they were alone with either parent. There are many pressures and many distractions to contend with, and it is often easier to give "presents" than our presence. However, your own focused attention is the best way for your child to feel genuinely and deeply loved for himself. And this feeling will be the primary basis for his development as a person.

Finally, it should be mentioned that accepting a child unconditionally does not mean condoning all his behavior or never setting limits. Far from it. What it does mean is accepting a child at each moment as the "best possible" child he can be at that moment. Limits can be set, misbehavior can be managed, and we can respond to whatever needs to be dealt with. But these things can be done without blame or judgment of the child's character.

Eye Contact, Physical Contact, and Words of Love

Also extremely important in communicating love and unconditional acceptance to children are appropriate use of eye contact and physical affection. Many parents use eye contact primarily when disciplining the child rather than as a way of establishing connection with and expressing love to a child. Using eye contact to convey our interest in relating to the child is extremely useful when we want to communicate our positive messages of love and caring.

Children also thrive on appropriate physical affection. Although the manner in which it is expressed changes, physical affection can be as important for adolescents as it is for babies. In fact, the famous family therapist, Virginia Satir, has said that children, teenagers, and even adults need two hugs per day for survival, six for maintenance, and twelve for growth!

Telling children in every conceivable way that they are loved and treasured is also important. Review their special or unique qualities and let them know that you will love them no matter what. Young children particularly enjoy games designed to convey the message of unconditional love. For example, children love it when a parent says, "Let's think of all the things you could do that would make me love you less than one million percent." Playful exploration of this question inevitably leads to the reassurance that nothing a child could do or say would reduce a parent's love.

Research has shown that the last thirty minutes before sleep are particularly "impressionable" periods, as the brain "replays" material from this period many more times than the material from other times during the day. Use this period to tell your child of his specialness and your love for him. The importance of this time also suggests the wisdom of minimizing bedtime arguments and struggles.

A Climate of Safety

In addition to expressions of unconditional love through focused attention, eye contact, physical affection, and words of love, Dorothy Corkille Briggs has written that children require a "climate of safety" in order to feel deeply loved. This climate of safety involves the following:

1. Trust based on honesty in the relationship.
2. Non-judgment—which means that we do not blame or attack our children's personal worth.
3. Cherishing our children as unique.
4. "Owning" our own feelings and respecting that our children have their own feelings which can be different from ours without making them wrong.

5. Empathy, which communicates that we care enough to try to understand things from their point of view.
6. Respect for your child's "unique growing" –acknowledging his natural urge to grow in the direction of self-sufficiency.Working on developing this kind of climate will help to ensure a strong basis for personality development.

A Sense of Belonging

Another important aspect of helping your child feel loved is helping him feel that he is connected with and belongs to his family, community, school, church, synagogue, or mosque, and the human race.

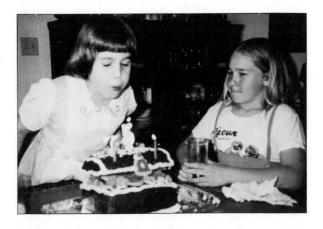

If a child feels that he does not really fit in and has trouble finding a place for himself, he will have doubts about his own worth and about his ability to find his own way. There are at least four key elements in helping a child feel that he is an important member of the family.

Share Yourself

Sharing your feelings, within appropriate limits, with your children helps them feel "connected" to you and more a part of your life. Share your interests and your hobbies with your child, and let him know that his interests are valued as well. Provide ample opportunities for the family members to work and play together. In this way your child can feel that he belongs to and is able to contribute to something larger than himself.

Strengthen Family Ties

First, keep a picture of the whole family by your child's bed where he can view it before falling asleep and upon awakening. In this way, he can *see* during these impressionable times that he is a part of a family and that he has a place. It is also helpful to teach children about their own past and about yours. Children love to hear stories about when they (and you) were little and to see pictures from their (and your) past. This fosters their connection with their parents and their heritage. Setting family goals is also a way of helping children feel that they contribute to the family.

Set Rules and Regulations That Emphasize Family Unity

Set rules to limit arguing and fighting. Be authoritative in enforcing rules about how family members speak to and treat each other. Insist that, "In this family we do not criticize each other" or, "In this family we build each other up, not tear each other down." Also, develop procedures for resolving conflict. Many families find the "family council" recommended by Rudolf Dreikurs in his book, *Children the Challenge*, to be very useful for this purpose.

Give Your Child His Own Space

Your child should have his own physical space even if it is only a shelf or a corner of a room shared with a sibling. Decisions about what to keep in this space or how to keep it should be made by him. He should also have his own seat at the table, so that there will be an obvious "hole" if he misses a meal.

Children with epilepsy also need help belonging to or fitting into social groups, classrooms, or athletic teams. They need help dealing with the perception of being different. It is important to teach children skills for social competence and to "coach" them on contributing to groups and activities of various kinds.

When a child comes home unhappy or discouraged about his difficulty participating in a group, I have found that it is best to first listen and to let the child know that you are trying to understand his feelings. At the same time, it is important that parents not "buy into" a child's perception that a situation is "awful" or "horrible." When a child feels sorry for himself, it is important that parents acknowledge his sadness but let the child know clearly that they do not feel sorry for him. The child needs to know that no matter how hopeless or discouraged he may be, you have confidence in him and his ability to handle his life. Eleanor Roosevelt once said, "No one can make you feel inferior without your permission." This is an important concept to get across to your child. For children who tend to focus on negative events, I frequently recommend that they keep a log each day of positive things that happen. I usually have the children start off at the end of the day by noting three or four things that went well. These things can be recorded on paper or a child can use a tape recorder. After a week at this level, I recommend that the child move up to four, five, six, and more positive things each day. When a child keeps track of positive things, it becomes more difficult to focus on negative events. This idea works great for adults too. In fact, parents and children keeping this kind of log together is very effective.

"I Am Capable"

For a child to feel capable he needs to feel a sense of responsibility. A child with a high sense of competence has a low need to control others. To foster a sense of responsibility:

Teach Choice

Make sure that your child learns personal responsibility. Teach him that his actions contribute to outcomes and that what he does makes a difference. Even fairly young children can be helped to realize that they are continually choosing to behave in one way or another and that their choices have consequences. Giving them a reasonable set of choices about how things are done will facilitate this process. Help them become aware of how they make decisions and how their choosing could be improved. This does not need to be done in an "I told you so" or "it's your own fault" manner. When a child chooses poorly, we can gently say "I'm sorry you chose... next time you may want to consider... "

Teach your child that life generally does not "happen to him" but rather that life is a "do-it-yourself" proposition. This can be a difficult lesson for children with epilepsy, as they often wonder why epilepsy happened to them or why God "chose" them to have seizures.

However, it is crucial for them to understand that with most things, the way they think, feel, and behave makes an important difference.

Perhaps most importantly, teach him that he is responsible for what he feels. While children should be encouraged to express their feelings directly and appropriately, they can learn little by little to avoid blaming others for their feelings. Parents should resist taking on their child's problems as their own.

Several of the books and audiotape programs listed at the end of the book will be helpful in knowing how to introduce the idea of emotional responsibility to children.

Teach Social Competence

Teach your child how to influence others in a positive way. Be sure to model and insist upon good manners. Good manners are particularly important for children with any kind of developmental or health problems, as they reduce the risk of further stigma or social rejection. Role playing can be useful for teaching appropriate social behavior. If your child resists role playing with you, he may be willing to practice with an older brother or sister. Allow your child as much as possible to solve his own problems (with your guidance), rather than solving them for him. It will also be helpful to teach him to be reasonably assertive: help your child learn to stand up for himself by expressing his needs and desires clearly and by voicing disagreement without apology.

Teach the Importance of Participation and Earning One's Keep

Involve your child in significant decisions that affect him. This will not only foster his sense of belonging to the family but also will enhance his sense of power. To help children learn responsibility, be sure that everyone contributes to the family in his own way. Even a toddler can be given chores like carrying the wastebasket to the door. Young children often enjoy having a list of their "chores" posted in the kitchen and experience great satisfaction in contributing to the family. Being able to work for or toward something they want, and thereby *earn* it, contributes enormously to helping children learn responsibility.

Once a child is capable of doing a task, give him the opportunity to do it. Another way of saying this is "never do for a child what he can do for himself." There are exceptions to this, for instance, when a child is sick or tired, but it is generally a good guideline. Helping your child become as independent and self-sufficient as possible will greatly increase his sense of competence. Minimizing the amount of a child's television viewing also fosters competence, as a child must rely more heavily on his own imagination and resourcefulness.

Facilitate the Experience of Success

Being successful fosters a sense of competence. Plan your child's activities so that he is likely to experience small steps of success. Difficult tasks can be broken into small steps with help and encour-

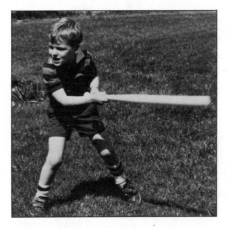

agement offered as needed. Focus on his strengths and aptitudes. Become aware of any specific talents he displays and provide opportunities to pursue and develop them.

Children should be encouraged to take on increasingly challenging tasks and responsibilities and (within limits) to "take risks." For the parent of a child with seizures, however, knowing what is appropriate risk taking and what is simply flirting with danger is difficult; knowing how to encourage appropriate risk-taking without putting your child's health in jeopardy takes courage and experience. It is important to try to include your child in all sports and activities of interest to him. If medically restricted, it is wise to try to find a way to modify an activity to allow at least partial participation. Of particular importance is remaining available to discuss these situations with your child and staying open to reconsidering the situation with his physician on a periodic basis.

Avoid Criticism, Comparison, and Competition

Destructive criticism cripples children more than physical handicaps. Period. Criticism and ridicule make children feel that their own approach to things is not respected. Furthermore, criticism is almost never effective in improving behavior and almost always leads to feelings of anger and resentment. Parents are often far more critical of their children, and each other, than they are of almost anyone else. The saying that "if parents treated their friends like they treated their children they would not have any friends" is too often true. This does not mean that parents should not point the way to better behavior or be firm in discipline. It simply means that there are more effective ways to accomplish these things than through criticism.

Comparing a child with others is also often harmful as it devalues a child's own efforts. The use of competition to motivate children should also be avoided, as it frequently breeds feelings of inferiority in the loser and guilt in the winner. A strong sense of competitiveness is not necessary for a sense of power. In fact, research has demonstrated that successful people are not highly competitive in the sense of having a strong need to beat the other guy. They are highly interested in challenging activity and enjoy hard work, but they are not inordinately motivated by a need to win.

Respect Your Child's Uniqueness

Look for and acknowledge ways in which your child has a different or special approach to a task. Respect your child as an individual person who from birth has his own predispositions and personality. Always consider him as an independent person who has real feelings of his own, and encourage him to express his feelings and ideas when they are different from others'. Teach him that there has never been, and will never be, another person exactly like him, that he is unique and therefore special.

Children also have unique interests, and it is generally wiser to try to understand and encourage these than to try to change them. Encouraging a child to keep a list of the things he wants helps to foster appreciation for his own desires and interests. A personal diary can become his record of his own story. Young children can dictate to their parents. Scrapbooks, bulletin boards, and a box for collecting private things also help nurture a sense of specialness.

Pity, Overprotection, and Dependency

For parents of children with serious medical conditions and significant handicaps, fostering a sense of capability is extremely challenging. It is still possible, of course, to help even an extremely impaired youngster feel that he has unique qualities and that he can do many things competently. However, the dependency on their parents can make developing a sense of power and responsibility very difficult. Many youngsters with seizures do in fact need far more attention than do most other children. In the context of this dependent relationship, every attempt should be made to allow the child to do for himself, and much should be made of even small steps toward independence.

When an appropriate dependent relationship develops between a parent and a child, it is often hard for the child and parent to give up the familiar routines when they no longer necessary. I have worked with parents who continued to dress their eight- or nine-year-old children long after the need to do so had passed. It is important to recognize this tendency and to remember that for high self-esteem, a child needs to experience as much independence and self-sufficiency as he can. Help can be adjusted in at least two ways: you can offer to help after your child has tried the task on his own; you can offer to help during part of an activity only. "You get started and I'll help with the buttons."

To really foster independence in a child with epilepsy, it is crucial to minimize or eliminate pity for the child and for oneself. There is little that is more crippling to a child than being felt sorry for. When a child feels pitied, he feels that his condition really must be terrible and feels discouraged about himself. A child with epilepsy understandably has many fears about his condition and how it will affect his life. This does not mean, however, that anyone needs to feel sorry for him. A child with epilepsy needs a courageous attitude toward life, which is obviously undermined by pity. If a parent can move toward accepting the child's situation and his feelings without pity, but rather with courage and faith in the child's ability to handle his difficulties, the child will be greatly helped.

Motivation, Praise, and Encouragement

Self-esteem and motivation are very closely related, and because a child's motivation to develop his abilities and perform well is so important, it will be given special attention here. The area of motivation is one in which the convictions of being lovable and being capable overlap. For a child to be motivated to learn, he has to believe that his own self-worth does not ride on never making mistakes, and he must believe that he has the ability to develop his own competence and skills.

Over the last ten years, Dr. Carol Dweck at the University of Illinois has studied motivational patterns in children. Two distinct motivational patterns have been identified on the basis of her research, an *adaptive* pattern and a *maladaptive* one. The adaptive pattern is characterized by a preference for challenging tasks and increased effort when things become difficult. Children who demonstrate this pattern typically focus on the *process* of developing their skills, knowledge, and competence. The maladaptive pattern is characterized by preference for easy tasks and a tendency to give up in the face of challenge. Children with this pattern focus on either gaining a positive judgment of their competence or avoiding a negative judgment. In other words, the children with the maladaptive motivational patterns are preoccupied with their own adequacy and strongly resist taking the risks necessary for optimal learning and performance. High self-esteem, which requires an inner conviction of one's worth independent of performance, clearly is the basis for a more adaptive motivational pattern.

The implications of this research for parents are several. First, focus on self-esteem, fostering these important convictions to help your child develop an adaptive motivational pattern. Second, it is wise for parents to focus on the *process* of a child's performance and not be preoccupied with the *product*. Turning our attention to our children's interests, efforts, and improvements helps to reduce the likelihood that they will come to equate their own worth with the quality of their performance or product.

Third, teach satisfaction with small gains – use the analogy that mountain climbers take one slow step at a time to accomplish mind-boggling feats. Fourth, use praise descriptively, not to evaluate children or their work. For many children, evaluative praise such as, "You're such a smart boy;" "What a beautiful painting," is very motivating and reinforces their sense of competence and worthiness. However, not all children find this kind of praise encouraging, and, in fact, many distrust it. Some children doubt their own abilities, and being told that they are smart or have produced a beautiful painting causes them to question the sincerity, or the critical judgment, of the praiser. It might be better, in this case, to say "I like the colors you chose in your painting."

Discipline

The way a child is disciplined strongly influences the development of his self-esteem. Loving discipline, in which the child is treated with patience, kindness, and reason rather than anger, criticism, humiliation, or harsh punishment, is a very powerful tool for developing self-esteem, as it fosters a sense of being respected and cared about. Discipline is really a means of *teaching* a child to be successful in life – that is, teaching a child what behavior works in this world and what does not.

There are many effective systems of discipline that are useful for helping a parent: 1) determine what is appropriate and inappropriate behavior and 2) determine appropriate consequences for behavior. An effective system of discipline allows parents to let children know that they "mean what they say," without continually criticizing or threatening. This advice works equally well for influencing children and adults. Becoming a master of discipline will help you stay as positive as possible with your child.

Children with epilepsy can pose more disciplinary problems for parents than children without. Sometimes the seizures themselves cause aggressive, anti-social, or difficult behavior. Other times the seizures contribute to problems of paying attention and following directions, which can be caused by medication as well. This simply underscores the importance of becoming a master of discipline. Learning the many alternatives to punishment can be particularly useful. See particularly the books by Rudolf Dreikurs, Adele Faber, and Elaine Mazlish in the Reading List.

PART II: YOUR SELF-ESTEEM

Your Self-Esteem Affects Your Child's

One of the most powerful ways you can help your child is to build your own self-esteem. Parents with low self-esteem tend to have trouble building esteem in their children for several reasons. They may attempt to live "through" their children, be self-critical and overly critical of the child, be threatened by a child's or teenager's desire for independence, hold negative expectations about life, or have trouble focusing on a child's strengths, rather than his weaknesses.

Parents as Mirrors and Models

Parents are both mirrors and models for their children. This means that parents reflect (through their reactions) to their children images of their acceptability and worth. Many experts believe that babies are born without any sense of self or identity at all. That is, while human beings are born with various temperamental predispositions to respond to the environment in certain ways, they do not have any kind of clear picture of themselves as separate beings; they will learn who they are through the way the environment and their parents respond to them. The child who sees that he produces enjoyment, love, and joy in his parents comes to see that he is an enjoyable, lovable, and joy-producing person. In this way, parents are mirrors for their developing children.

Parents also model self-esteem (high or low) for their children. They do this through their behavior and their attitudes. By observing their parents, children observe how grown-ups respect themselves, care for themselves, and treat others. They also learn how adults approach life.

The Choice of High Self-Esteem

Parents of children with epilepsy have several additional challenges to developing and/or maintaining their own self-esteem. The emotional and financial strain and the increased likelihood that both parents will, at least at times, be fatigued pose a challenge to high esteem and to keeping life in perspective. Also, having a child with epilepsy can assault a parent's esteem by triggering excessive worry, embarrassment (especially if the child is handicapped in observable ways), and guilt. The challenge of never having consistent expectations—as the course of epilepsy is so unpredictable—further makes planning ahead very difficult and undermines a sense of control and capability.

However, the parent of a child with epilepsy—like any parent—may choose high self-esteem at any time. That is, for adults, high self-esteem begins with *a decision*—that I am lovable and capable as I am, even though I am not perfect and even if others do not think so. This decision is necessary for high self-esteem and, in my judgement, is the hallmark of maturity. However, it takes considerable courage, energy, and work to put into practice. No one "confers" high esteem on grown-ups; it must be claimed and accepted.

To parents of youngsters with very difficult seizures and/or secondary handicaps, it may sound selfish to focus on their own self-esteem and not on the child's needs. Many parents wonder, "How could I be happy and at ease when my child has so many problems, suffers so much, and has such a hard life?" However, it is always the case that parents are most helpful to their children with problems when they themselves feel calm, self-satisfied, and happy. If parents get stuck in their own negative emotions, they are unable to attend effectively to all the little things which, totaled together, have a big effect on their child's life. Furthermore, if parents do not choose to grow in the direction of increasing happiness and self-esteem *regardless* of the child's condition, the child is then put in the position of feeling responsible for his parent's state of happiness or unhappiness. This is an inappropriate responsibility for a child. The importance of "working on yourself" thus cannot be over-emphasized, especially considering that a negative self-image usually becomes increasingly negative with age unless challenged and reworked.

Many adults also have a deep distrust of the rightness of self-esteem, believing that unless they are perfect they should not accept and love themselves as they are. Despite the fact that when we have high self-esteem we are not an emotional burden on others, we often need some convincing that it is all right for us to choose high self-esteem. Determining our level of self-worth is up to us. Deciding that you are lovable and worthwhile as you are may be the most important and useful decision you could ever make.

Acceptance of Yourself, Warts and All

The decision for high self-esteem is in part a decision to accept yourself as you are, right now, or as Shakespeare said, "warts and all."

This means three things:

1. Accepting yourself exactly as you are, even though you are not perfect and want to be better.

2. Forgiving yourself completely for all the foolish, wicked, brainless, hurtful things you have done. Forgiveness means to let go—to not be influenced any more by the restrictive pull of the past; it is something we do to free ourselves to become better people.

3. Continuing to accept yourself each moment of each day as you develop more and more into the person you would like to become.

Parents of children with epilepsy often face enormous challenges in the area of acceptance, particularly acceptance of painful feelings like anger or guilt. When your feelings are accepted, they are more easily changed or given up altogether. Parents who deny or hang onto these feelings suffer needlessly and are ineffective.

Parents need to be able to express their feelings to others without the fear of being criticized as a bad or rejecting parent. Sometimes this safety is available with a spouse or relative, or with a friend. Sometimes it is necessary to find this safety in a "neutral" counselor whose job it is to listen to and help understand feelings without judgment.

"Reprogramming" for High Self-Esteem

Once you have chosen high esteem, you need to work on changing the years of negative programming that kept you at lower-than-optimal levels of esteem. In some cases psychotherapy may be necessary to support the changes in thinking, believing, and feeling that you want to make. Claiming high self-esteem usually involves uncovering, examining, and discarding unproductive beliefs about ourselves and the world and replacing them with more useful beliefs.

PART III: THE ASSERTIVE PARENT

Assertiveness, Active Coping, and High Self-Esteem

There is much talk these days about "empowering" parents to deal with the professionals and the bureaucracies that serve their children. A sense of personal power and a sense of competence are necessary for high self-esteem, and these can be developed through acting assertively and through holding positive expectations. Those parents who have been able to raise their handicapped or chronically ill children with success and joy have usually educated themselves about their child's conditions and their rights, as you are now doing by reading this book. Knowledge is power, and my practice is full of examples of people who have used this power assertively to the great benefit of their children. Several suggestions may be useful regarding being appropriately assertive and holding positive expectations:

1. *Question authority, even if it is a doctor.* It is your right to know about the medical, developmental, educational, and social status of your child. Expect answers; "push" reluctant professionals when necessary. Be a part of the treatment plan. Be aware that the goal for your child is optimal services.

2. *Don't be bossed around by statistics.* That is, if the doctor says there is a ten to one chance of having a particular problem, you have every right to assume and expect that your child will be the one in ten who does not have the problem. We know from an extremely large number of research studies that the expectations we hold for ourselves and for others strongly affect what happens. While parents need to get whatever help is necessary for their child and to make all reasonable plans for the future, it is emotionally right and scientific to expect positive outcomes for your child.

3. *If unsatisfied with professional help, change doctors.* At least two or three times per month I hear a story in my office of a parent who was told something untrue or unkind by a profes-

sional and how changing professionals made a world of difference.

4. *Trust your instincts.* Many times parents intuitively know that something is right or wrong for their child and are not taken seriously. Often only through the parent's insistence is a child properly diagnosed, taken off an inappropriate medication, or given a needed educational service. It is at times imperative that you keep on insisting, especially when you are sure that you know your child best.

Living In The Here And Now, One Day At A Time

People living with a wide variety of conditions from alcoholism to cancer have found the most helpful perspective on living to be taking life one day at a time. Given the degree of uncertainty that parents of children with epilepsy face, this is probably "the perspective of choice" for you as well. Take it one day at a time and try to focus on the small steps you accomplish each day. For many parents, the tendency to worry about their child's future is so strong that living in the present and taking one day at a time are very difficult. These parents spend a lot of time imagining the feared future. They have difficulty making decisions because they are fearful that if they choose incorrectly they will regret the decision for the rest of their lives. I often point out to parents that they will only regret a decision the rest of their lives if they *choose* to constantly compare the way things turned out with their *fantasy* about what might have been. This emphasis on choice is very useful to parents, and many come to believe that they have enormous power to choose to appreciate *what is*, rather than constantly compare the present to what might have been. A related issue is what I call the "fear of getting stuck," which I believe underlies many of the problems of modern life. For example, marriages are inclined to break up not so much on the basis of the problems the partners may have but on the basis of at least one partner's fear that "I'm going to have to live with this the rest of my life." This fear of getting stuck paralyzes an individual and keeps him from dealing with life as it is, one day at a time. It also prohibits the recognition that people can and do change.

The Role of Beliefs

In my experience, parents of a child with medical or developmental problems frequently hold the deep belief that if they did not worry about the child's future, they would not do the things that need to be done to ensure the best possible future for their child. Uncovering and evaluating such beliefs is extremely important for learning to live happily in the here and now.

I recently had a very dramatic counseling session with the parents of a nineteen-year-old boy with epilepsy and developmental difficulties. His mother explained that for years she had experienced extreme anxiety about the boy's future and what would happen to him if he were not able to live independently when the parents die. I questioned her about the beliefs that lay underneath her anxiety. What she revealed was the belief described above—that if she did not worry constantly about her son, she would not take care of whatever needed to be taken care of to ensure his future. When asked if she would not take care of these things simply out of love for her boy, she replied that of course she would. She then wept and eventually laughed at the realization that worry and anxiety were not necessary to motivate her to be a good mother.

Many related beliefs contribute to parents' emotional upset such as "If I didn't worry constantly I might not appreciate the extent of my child's needs." However, in my experience almost every parent can learn that simply on the basis of love for the child, he can do whatever is necessary for his child. Most parents report that they are more caring and loving when they are happy with (and not sorry for or anxious about) their child.

Going Beyond Coping

Many parents of youngsters with epilepsy experience a level of physical, emotional, and financial challenge almost inconceivable to parents of children without seizures, and life can be at times almost overwhelming. While pity, false optimism, and homilies typically are not useful for such parents, it is helpful to know that there is light at the end the tunnel. And, as incredible as it seems, parents do cope with such problems, and many experience abundant joy, satisfaction, and gratitude to boot. No matter how devastating circumstances may have been, they have moved forward. However, these parents have had to *claim* the right to be happy, to be proud of their children and themselves. It is not granted by others. The question is not whether you can experience the gamut of joy and satisfaction with your youngster who has epilepsy, but how soon you get on with the process.

The world is full of parents who, after the initial shock and grief of the diagnosis of epilepsy, have come to find that their child with epilepsy has enriched their lives to such an immeasurable extent that they no longer wish that he was different, nor would they trade him for a "normal" child. While they hope for a cure, they do not continually lament that the child is not "normal." Although they do everything in their power to help the child live as normally and happily as possible, they do not continue to wish that something that did happen had not happened. They avoid self-pity, with its destructive effects, and they resist the subtle message from others that there is something "wrong" with their child and that they must be devastated. They assert that this is their child whom they love more than anything else in the world and whose many wonderful qualities they cherish.

One of the statements that I recommend to parents to help develop high self-esteem is, "I'd rather be me than anyone else." Parents who thrive with their challenging children have a related attitude: that they would rather have their child be as he is than be anyone else.

Getting to a position of acceptance and joy is a gradual process, but it can happen. You can go far beyond coping with a difficult problem; you can thrive. Perhaps most incredible, many parents have described ways in which their child with epilepsy has enriched family life. Because of their youngster with seizures, parents have had extraordinary opportunities to develop the qualities of patience, devotion, love, and a sense of humor, while siblings have become more sensitive than they may have otherwise been to the needs of others, particularly those who are in some ways different from the norm.

As unbelievable as it sounds, children too can come to see the silver lining in the cloud of epilepsy. Some have pointed to the way in which being on antiepileptic medication kept them from experimenting with dangerous drugs which badly damaged the lives of others in their peer group. This is a great task for the rest of our life – to develop an appreciative and grateful attitude for everything in life, and it is a great task to try to instill this attitude in our children. This may seem like too much for right now. But I believe you can get there.

Parent Statements

It's been so hard to watch him with all these setbacks. Last year when the kids made National Honor Society or got academic letters he came home almost in tears. That would have been him if this wouldn't have happened.

You have to live this way and make a conscious decision to keep on living as if nothing were wrong. I wrote a letter to his camp, where he'll be going this summer, about his self-esteem and how they shouldn't bother him. He's going white water rafting. We don't know if he's pushing limits to see how far he can go or to prove that he's just like everybody else. I just don't know. Or maybe he is the one who doesn't think twice about his epilepsy, we do, and he's going because he wants to go white water rafting, and that's all.

There was a lot of ambivalence on my part. Do I like her, don't I like her? Do I love her, don't I? I'm going to have a baby for the rest of my life. I wanted a baby but I wanted her to grow. She's still in diapers and she's not walking yet and she's heavy. All those feelings. Can I stand this?

His sister is really good for him because I hurt so much for him that my tendency is to overprotect him. On the other hand, she treats him like a normal brother.

Sometimes I think that Stephen thinks his problems are more psychological than due to the epilepsy. He has a tendency to blame himself for his problems not realizing that most of them are caused by the epilepsy.

He's done some wonderful things. When he's had to do special projects, speaking projects at school, he's always done them on epilepsy, with no prompting from us. He's been doing this since 9th grade. He's trying to explain to other kids what it's like. Part of him is withdrawn and part is trying to reach out and explain and say, "I'm just like you except I have this problem and this is what causes it."

In a way all parents of needy children somehow find the strength from within to care and provide for their kids. I never thought I'd think this way, it's kind of trite but so real.

I walked away from the neurologist feeling like I had been rolled over by a steam roller. I got myself scraped up only to find myself flattened again. Each time the hope is diminished, the light is getting dimmer and dimmer. But what can they do? I don't want them to give me false hope.

I don't think we've lost any friends because of Matthew's handicap. I would say however that I don't know what to do in a lot of social situations or for his social life. I think I'm limiting us because I don't know how to act socially. It's a problem for us. His peers sometimes reject him. He stumbles, he drools, and wears a helmet.

Our son's epilepsy has really affected our sense of self-esteem. We've both gained weight in the past two years. We've literally stayed home, watching and waiting for the next tragedy. It's just now that we're starting to come out and go on with our lives.

I always feel socially inept. Life didn't tell me what I was supposed to do in this situation. I'm not exactly sure what to say to people.

One coping mechanism is just taking it day by day, however, that is one of the frustrations, the inability to plan. You can plan all you feel like but then your child has a bad day and it's all down the tubes. That phrase taking it one day at a time never had much meaning for me although it does now.

My advice to parents is that the pain will go away, not completely, you'll always feel sad, but you will feel better. One day you will wake up and the skies will be blue and it'll be a nice day. Your child will be ill but that will be a part of it. It doesn't negate the fact that life is nice.

We try to let all our kids know that if anything serious happened to them, we'd fight with everything we had in us and not turn our backs on them. That is a very good feeling for kids to have in these days and times.

One of the most important things is to get feedback from your child. Don't make any assumptions about what they understand.

My daughter's very smart and the other kids think that that's the reason she spells so well, because she has this extra electricity in her brain!

The neurosurgeon who first took care of our child told us there was a lot of misunderstanding about people with epilepsy. He also sat us down and told us the most important thing you must do is to treat this child normally. He went on and on about how important it was. We've really taken his advice. I'm not sure how we would have treated him without that doctor's advice.

Our son has tonic/clonic seizures. Right now he's two miles in a cave spelunking. He rappels down 65 foot stone cliffs. He plays soccer, rides his bike all over the place, and does anything he wants to.

I think self-esteem is the most important thing I can help do for my child. If he only feels good about himself, that's all that matters to me. How can he succeed at anything if he has a low opinion of himself?

We've sought psychological counseling because of Kirsten's be-

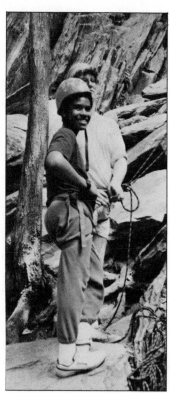

havior. She really gets temperamental and out of control. The group experience helped so much. Just to hear that we weren't alone in all this.

To me, acceptance is the key word. Learning to accept that your life is going to be different than you'd imagined, more difficult than you'd imagined. Do a lot of reading, ask a lot of questions, and trust yourself and what you observe. The doctors don't know everything.

I don't think anyone's life should be reduced to the label of being an epileptic. It denies all the other facets of that person's life.

We really try to build self-esteem in our kids but seizures have a way of causing sadness. Sometimes it's so hard to see past the sadness.

Even though we have the sweetest, most lovable child around, he's very demanding and requires constant care and attention. We feel chronically drained. How can we send positive messages?

We love that little boy more than anything. Everyone in the family smiles at him, kisses him, hugs him, claps for him. We let him know when he's made an achievement with a standing ovation. No matter what he grows up to be, he'll have all his family here, loving him. And when we're gone, he'll find courage and strength from our love.

SIX

When Epilepsy Is Not The Only Problem . . . Assessing Special Needs

PATRICIA QUINN, M.D.*

The child with seizures has many faces. She can be a tiny infant just two days old, or a boy who developed infantile spasms at three months of age. He can be a three year old who suddenly starts having seizures at night, or a five year old with generalized tonic/clonic seizures. He can be a child with cerebral palsy who has epilepsy as well, or a child with an unknown neurological impairment and uncontrolled seizures. Epilepsy is a condition with a variety of symptoms as well as intellectual and behavioral manifestations. There is usually no set course of treatment and no true range of expectations that we physicians can provide for parents. Each child responds to treatments in unique and unpredictable ways and is a constant challenge to researchers and diagnosticians.

As parents of children with epilepsy, you want to know all there is to know and to do all that you can for your children. This chapter is directed toward families with children who have epilepsy as well as special needs. There are many children who live quite normal lives for

---

* Patricia Quinn is a developmental pediatrician in the Washington, D.C. area.

whom epilepsy is an inconvenience more than a disability. I don't wish to diminish the shattering experience of a diagnosis of epilepsy for those children and families. However, there are many children who have to contend not only with epilepsy but with a variety of other handicaps.

Until recently our society has left a large segment of special needs children in the shadows. In the last fifteen years giant strides have been made toward recognizing the need to change society's attitudes toward disabled people. Because of the efforts of parents and advocates, we

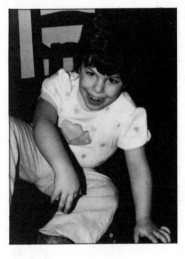

now have the legal framework established to help children reach their potential. Not only have public buildings been made more accessible but the educational system has created programs to assess and meet the educational rights of children with special needs.

But how do you get your child integrated into that system? This chapter and Chapter 7 will answer that question. But first of all you will need to determine a course of action, and act upon it immediately if your child is to benefit. I have seen denial destroy children, parents, and families.

Inaction can complicate the picture for years to come with a possibly poorer long term outcome. My own experience as the parent of a child with epilepsy is that the sooner you act, the better.

> *I first noticed jerks in my nine-month-old daughter that I immediately recognized as infantile spasms on a Friday night. As a developmental pediatrician, I knew all the implications of this diagnosis at once. At that point, I so wished I was wrong but couldn't deny what I was observing. After observing more spasms on Saturday, I called a pediatric neurologist and my daughter had her first EEG on Monday morning. Treatment options were discussed, I read most of the current literature, and a decision was made as to the course of treatment within 72 hours of my first*

observation. For the next four months she continued to have spasms and her developmental progress slowed. She was monitored closely neurologically and developmentally. She received intervention (speech therapy) and now at age four is progressing well.

As a parent I can speak to the feelings and as a professional, I can speak to the critical need for early recognition and prompt treatment in order to get the best possible developmental outcome for your child. The first step in this process is understanding more about "normal" development.

This chapter describes what development is, how epilepsy can affect development, what "special needs" means, how to get your child assessed, the role of the developmental pediatrician, and other developmental considerations.

What Is "Development?"

Human development is a miraculous and complex process of maturing and acquiring skills. Every child's development is different because of a unique genetic background and environment. There is a wide range of what is considered "normal" development, and each child has his own individual developmental profile. This section reviews what development is and how epilepsy can affect your child's development.

The Areas of Development

Although all areas of development are interrelated and should be assessed as a whole, development in young children is usually assessed in six areas: 1) gross motor; 2) fine motor; 3) cognition; 4) language; 5) social; and 6) self-help. These terms are used frequently; some working definitions follow:

Gross Motor. Gross motor development involves the use of the body's large muscles, such as the legs, arms, and abdomen. Sitting, crawling, and walking are gross motor skills.

Fine Motor. Fine motor skills involve the use of the body's small muscles, such as the hands and fingers. In addition, control of eye and mouth muscles are fine motor skills. Typical fine motor activities include drawing and eating.

Cognition. Cognitive ability is the ability of a child to think, reason, and analyze. Its exact definition and measurement have been the subject of debate for many years.

Language. Communication is central to child development, and the use of language involves two types of communication. Receptive language is the ability to understand gestures, words, and symbols. Expressive language is the ability to use gestures, words, and symbols to communicate with others.

Social. Social development is the ability to function in relation to other people. How a child plays with other children, interacts with adults, and asserts his independence are all social skills.

Self-Help. Learning how to take care of oneself is an important area of development. Children usually progress from total dependence on their parents to being able to take care of themselves. Dressing, feeding, and toileting are all important self-help skills.

Sensory integration is often considered a separate area of development, but it affects each of the other areas tremendously. Sensory integration involves the reception and processing of sensations such as sound, touch, light, movement, and smell. Children with epilepsy can suffer from sensory integration problems because seizures can interfere with their ability to receive and process these stimuli.

The Sequence Of Development

Parents of all children—but especially parents of children with epilepsy—are very interested in their child's development. Often parents' questions about childhood development center on when a child will learn a new skill like walking, talking, and writing. If you understand the sequence of development—the progression of learning skills—you will be able to put your child's progress into perspective. This knowledge can help you play a major role in assessing that progress. You, however, should always try to view your child's development as a complete picture and avoid preoccupation with any single area of development.

Figure 1 is a developmental checklist that shows the range of skills that are usually achieved by most children and the ages at which they are achieved. It provides a good guideline for what is considered "normal" development. Refer to it to get an idea of your child's developmental levels but do not use this guide as a developmental test or as a predictor of your child's future development.

Developmental Checklist *

Milestones Attained by 12 Months:

Social/Emotional

Gives objects on request

Imitates hand and face gestures such as waving "bye-bye," clapping hands, closing eyes

Helps with dressing by putting arms out for sleeves and feet for shoes

Seeks and finds hidden toys easily

Is affectionate toward familiar people

Motor (Fine)

Holds spoon but needs help with its use

Puts blocks in and out of a small box

Uses pincer grasp (thumb and index finger) to pick up small objects or pieces of food

Points with index finger toward desired objects

Uses both hands freely, but may demonstrate a preference for one

Motor (Gross)

Pulls to standing position and lets self down by holding onto furniture

May stand alone for a few seconds

Sits well for an indefinite period of time

May creep on all fours

May walk independently

---

* Reprinted from *Growing Child*, 22 North Second St., Lafayette, IN 47902

Communication

Imitates adult's playful sound making

Recognizes own name and turns to speaker when hearing it

Follows simple directions: "Give it to Mommy," "Come to Daddy," "Clap hands."

Vision

Recognizes familiar people at a distance of twenty feet or more

Watches intently small toys that are pulled across the floor at a distance of ten feet away

Milestones Attained by 18 Months:

Social/Emotional

Raises and holds cup with two hands

Drinks from a cup without spilling

Removes shoes, socks, cap

Imitates familiar actions such as sweeping floor, dusting, reading a book

Amuses self, but prefers to be near an adult

Alternates between independence and dependence on caregiver

Motor (Fine)

Scribbles with a crayon on paper

Can build a tower with three blocks after a demonstration

Picks up very small objects and food immediately on sight

Explores objects more frequently with hands than mouth

Motor (Gross)

Pushes and pulls large objects

Walks, but with feet slightly apart

Can do two things at once – carry a large object and walk with it

Climbs into a large chair, rotates body, and sits

May creep backward when going down stairs

Communication

Speaks six to twenty recognizable words

Likes nursery rhymes and joins in

Echoes the last word spoken to him/her

"Talks" to self while playing

Enjoys picture books

May point to two or three parts (eyes, nose, hair, shoes) on doll or self

Vision

Fixes eyes on and recovers a rolling ball ten feet away

Points to distant objects out of doors

Milestones Attained by 24 Months:

Social/Emotional

Uses a spoon to feed self

Chews food well

Raises and drinks from cup, then replaces it on table

Is very possessive about toys—no sharing

Plays beside but not with other children

Clings to caregiver when tired or afraid

Goes into tantrums when frustrated, but can be readily distracted

Demands a lot of caregiver's attention

Motor (Fine)

Removes wrapper from a cupcake or candy bar

Builds a tower of six blocks

Copies a vertical line with a crayon on paper

Turns pages in a book one at a time

Picks up tiny objects as small as a crumb

Motor (Gross)

Runs on whole foot, but can stop, start, and run around obstacles easily

Climbs stairs holding onto the railing (walks two feet to each step)

Pulls wheeled toy forward and backward by string

Throws a small ball

Walks into a large ball when intending to kick it

Communication

Engages in simple pretend play

Uses fifty or more recognizable words

Puts together two or more words to formulate a sentence

Asks "What's that?" constantly

Joins in nursery rhymes and songs

Refers to self by name

Points to and repeats the names of body parts such as eyes, nose, hair, feet, mouth

Understands simple commands and conversation

Milestones Attained by 36 Months:

Social/Emotional

Eats with spoon and fork

Washes hands, but needs supervision for drying

Dry during the day and often through the night

Plays with other children in and outdoors

Is affectionate toward younger children

Likes to help adults with chores

Pulls pants up and down, but can't button yet

Cooperates generally

Shares toys

Motor (Fine)

Builds a tower of nine blocks

Copies a bridge made with three blocks

Copies a circle with crayon on paper

Draws figure of a man which appears as a head with one or two features

Paints with large brush and paint

Closes fist and wiggles thumb (right or left)

Motor (Gross)

Alternates feet when walking up stairs (comes down with two feet to each step)

Rides tricycle

Walks on tiptoes

Stands on one foot momentarily when shown how

Jumps from bottom step of stairs

Communication

Gives full name, sex, age when asked

Asks questions "who," "what," "where?"

Enjoys listening to stories and wants favorite ones repeated over and over

Recites nursery rhymes

Uses plurals

Uses large vocabulary, but speech may contain misarticulations

Engages in a simple conversation

Talks about past experiences

Uses pronouns "I, me, you" correctly

Eager to talk about self and experiences with some stuttering not uncommon

Milestones Attained by 48 Months:

Social/Emotional

Eats well with fork and spoon

Dresses and undresses self except for laces, back buttons, and some snaps

Prefers companionship of other children to adults

Understands about taking turns

Motor (Fine)

Threads small beads if the needle is threaded first

Builds a tower of ten or more blocks

Holds and uses a crayon or pencil with good control

Copies an "O" (circle), " + " (plus), and "V"

Draws a house

Motor (Gross)

Can bend and touch toes without bending knees

Likes a variety of ball play

Runs on toes

Climbs, slides, swings actively

Walks skillfully on narrow line or cracks in sidewalk

Can stand on one foot (either foot) for eight seconds

Can hop forward (each foot) two yards

Communication

Tells connected stories of recent experiences

Can give name, address, and age (may show on fingers)

Asks questions constantly—"why, what, how, when?"

Knows several nursery rhymes and can repeat or sing them correctly

Counts by memory up to twenty

Enjoys jokes

Listens to and enjoys stories

Speaks grammatically and exhibits only a few sound substitutions (*r-l-w-y* group, *p-th-f-s* group or *k-t* group)

Milestones Attained by 60 Months:

Social/Emotional

Dresses and undresses independently

Uses knife and fork competently

Washes and dries hands and face well

Selects own playmates

Is protective toward younger children and animals

Comprehends rules of games and the concept of fair play

Demonstrates a sense of humor

Understands the necessity for tidiness, but requires frequent reminders

Experiences fears involving self – dogs, falling, physical dangers

Picks nose, bites nails

Sucks thumb only before falling asleep or when fatigued

Speech and Language

Speaks fluently except for a few mispronunciations *(s, v, f, th)*

Gives full name, age, birthday, address

Defines concrete words by their function

Asks meaning of abstract words and unfamiliar words and uses them subsequently

Loves to recite and chant jingles and rhymes

Enjoys being read to or told stories, and acts them out alone later

Visual-Motor Skills

Threads a large needle independently and sews real stitches

Copies circle, square, cross, and capital letters
V T H O X L Y U C A

Draws a house with these features: outline, door, windows, chimney, and roof

Draws a person with these features: head, arms, legs, trunk

Draws a variety of other items and names them *before* producing

Uses brush, crayons, and pencil with control

Crayons and colors forms within the lines

Matches ten colors

Names at least four primary colors

Copies block patterns containing ten blocks

Motor Development

Can walk a narrow line without stepping off.

Climbs, swings, runs skillfully.

Moves rhythmically to music.

Stands on one foot (either foot) with arms folded across chest to a count of ten seconds

Hops two to three yards forward on each foot

Enjoys ball play and understands rules, positions, and scoring

Bends and touches toes without bending knees

Grips strongly with each hand

Can run lightly on toes

Plateaus

All children have *plateau* (no change) periods as part of development. These are usually short, occur at the same time as rapid progress in another developmental area, and are followed by growth spurts. Babies, for instance, may learn fewer words or talk less as they begin to walk or explore. If your child enters a stage where no progress is seen for a prolonged period of time or if your child loses skills that she already has *(regresses)* it is important to act immediately to determine the reason. Are seizures under control? Are medication levels effective? Is the program appropriate? Has this been a period of prolonged medical illness, complications, and/or hospitalizations? Or is your child's condition getting worse? Contact your physician or neurologist to let him know of this change in your child's development.

Expectations and Development

As discussed below, epilepsy can affect your child's development. But as parents, you cannot afford to have epilepsy affect *your* developmental expectations for her. If you do – if you begin to believe that your child cannot learn certain skills – there is good chance her development *will* be hampered. Always expect your child to develop well or to get back on a good developmental track. Negative expectations can lead to self-fulfilling prophecies.

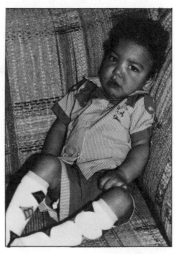

There is far more to achieving a developmental level than just how quickly a child learns a skill. *Quality*, not quantity, is the key. It is your job as a parent to provide opportunities for your child to learn, explore, and be curious. If a parent offers too little encouragement or steps in too often with help, development is hindered. Let your child take risks. It is far easier to comfort a child who has fallen while trying to climb than it is to stimulate an unmotivated child. Help your child learn a skill, and then let her do it herself.

If your child has been found to have delayed development, she will have "special needs" and require additional input and services to achieve to her potential.

What Does Special Needs Mean? Or What About Labeling?

Labels of all kinds are frequently attached to people or to groups. It is as simple a process as naming a child. Things must have names for identity purposes. For example, federal legislation provides money to school systems for their programs based on labels. Therefore, there must be classifications, but in dealing with children with epilepsy choosing your labels carefully is vital.

There are a variety of names we could use in this chapter and I will define each one now, although I will use "special needs" throughout.

Developmentally delayed or *disabled* refers to a child who progresses at a significantly slower rate than his peers in acquiring skills in the developmental areas discussed above. The disability can be attributed to a specific cause, occurs before age eighteen, and will probably continue throughout life. It may leave the person unable to function normally in society.

Multi-handicapped refers to a child who has two or more areas of impairment, such as a delay in gross motor and speech, and requires treatment of these impairments.

Special needs refers to a child who has developmental delays or is multi-handicapped and has needs that normal children do not have. Parents and professionals try to identify and provide programs to meet those special needs.

I urge parents to steer away from feeling obligated to limit their children to the strict definitions a label creates. To do so can lead to self-fulfilling prophecies. Sometimes a label can cause negative reactions if someone has outdated associations with words. After all, in the end, a label doesn't do anything for your child. It can actually be an ending rather than a beginning. Here the purpose of labeling is to place your child in an appropriate educational program and to determine the type of services she needs.

If your child has special needs, it is essential that you get a complete, accurate, and individualized picture of her in order to provide her with the specific services she needs. That is the goal of an assessment which is discussed in the next section.

Getting An Assessment

An individual assessment reveals who your child is with her strengths, weaknesses, and needs. During an assessment, all areas of your child's development should be examined closely. Just how this is done will vary for each child. Depending on when your child developed seizures, the type of assessment and the people assessing her will be different. If your child began having seizures during the first two years of life, it is absolutely critical that you act as soon as possible to obtain a developmental assessment so that intervention can be directed toward her areas of need and provide a baseline for measuring her development in the future. An accurate diagnosis is critical because the first two years are a time of rapid brain growth and change.

Who to Call for an Assessment

Hopefully your neurologist has already referred you to an appropriate agency or program run by the local school district. You can also turn to the yellow pages and find a developmental pediatrician, or call your own family physician for a referral. It is important to get "hooked up" with a program right now that will provide educational intervention for your child, and support for the family. The resource guide at the back of this book has addresses and phone numbers for parent advocacy organizations, state education departments, as well as toll free 800 numbers. Any of these can help you with any questions you have in getting an assessment referral.

The assessment is usually a coordinated effort of many people, and again, there are many labels for this team approach. But whatever the team calls itself, YOU are a member of that team. Your role as parent has become a widely recognized component of the team approach. Your observations and opinions about your child and her needs are valid. You know your child better than anyone else, you have spent more time with her, and can share information about her behavior in a variety of situations. For example, your child may attempt to talk and make noises at home that are not heard during an evaluation. This information is crucial to the assessment results. Your child's team can be made up of a number of different professionals. Figure 2 shows who is responsible for what.

The assessment will examine what skills your child possesses and whether she is behind, has lost skills, or is not gaining them at the rate she should. Children do not need to be taught certain skills in their early years because, as the brain matures, actions and reactions appear automatically. The child progresses automatically from one level to the next.

If a child does not have the skills he should have at a certain age, we say that he is delayed. By following a child and looking at how many

Figure 2. Areas of Development to be Assessed and Professionals Responsible for Each

AREA	SKILLS ASSESSED	SPECIALIST
Speech/Language	Articulation, pronunciation, verbal abilities, vocabulary, understanding and following directions	Speech Pathologist
Gross Motor	Using large muscles – walking skipping, running, throwing, balance & coordination	Physical Therapist
Fine Motor	Using small muscles – handwriting, buttoning, puzzles, eye tracking, feeding, hand dominance	Occupational Therapist
Perceptual/Sensory Processing	Visual perception, design copying, planning of body movements, and such skills as toleration of touch and movement in space necessary for sensory motor development	Occupational Therapist
Cognitive/Learning	IQ, learning styles, achievement, thinking, reasoning, understanding	Special Educator/Psychologist/ Educational Diagnostician
Hearing		Audiologist
Vision		Ophthalmologist/ Physician
Nutrition	Caloric intake, habits, variety of food, growth, nutritional status	Registered Dietician/Nutritionist
Medical	Brain maturation, related conditions	Pediatrician/ Developmental Pediatrician/ Neurologist
Social/Self Help	Family functioning, stresses, coping, dressing, feeding, sleeping, behaviors	Family worker/Social worker/Visiting teachers
Cognitive/ Learning – Drug Side-Effects	Sensory, perceptual and motor planning, detailed evaluation of affects on attention, memory, and sensory processing related to antiepileptic drugs	Neuropsychologist

skills he gains over certain time periods, we can evaluate his rate of progress. A child without problems will make six or more months of progress in six months and have a normal rate. If the rate of progress is slower, a child will still gain new skills, but will be behind other children at each point in time. For example, in the area of cognitive development, slower progress is what we call *retardation*. Degrees of retardation are based on how much progress is made over a certain time period. With severe retardation, there is little progress or change over time. With mild retardation, the child will be slower, but will have academic abilities. All areas of development should be assessed to determine where on the development scale your child currently falls.

As soon as possible after your child's epilepsy is diagnosed, it is important to obtain information about her developmental level. This is particularly important to determine if:

1. She is already behind.
2. She is continuing to make progress.
3. She is slowing down as a result of drug treatment or uncontrolled seizures.

It is important to follow your child over a period of time to monitor her progress, determine developmental levels, and intervene to help her learn the skills needed to progress to the next level.

Visiting the Developmental Pediatrician

When a child comes to be evaluated by a developmental pediatrician, several steps are taken to reach a diagnosis and establish a treatment plan. The developmental pediatrician can then act as a coordinator to help carry out that plan. An important part of the diagnosis of children with disabilities is the history. You will be asked questions about family backgrounds, illnesses, and about other family members with some of the same or similar symptoms as your child. Pregnancy and labor and delivery records are important, as are records of early developmental milestones such as walking, talking, and early social behavior. Previous test results, baby books, and pictures of your child during all stages of development are also significant. In addition, I request that parents bring samples of their child's school or art work done over the years and copies of all his report cards. All this background information helps establish, when possible, a cause or the time of onset of a child's disorder.

I also ask for a week-long diary, detailing the child's behaviors and parental interventions and interactions. This provides feedback on parenting and family needs. I also encourage parents to make a list of all concerns they may have or questions they would like answered.

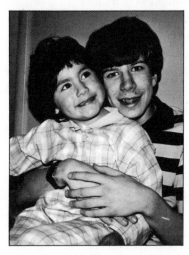

The next step is the interview with and examination of the child himself. Many children are very perceptive at describing difficulties they may have. Small children will be evaluated with the parents present, older children will be evaluated alone.

The neurodevelopmental examination consists of a series of tasks which the child will perform that allow us to look at brain functioning. Attention span, distractibility, and behaviors are all assessed during this session. Speech and language functioning—both *receptive* (what a child understands) and *expressive* (what a child says)—are evaluated. Hearing is tested. Memory and processing abilities are measured for visual, auditory, and tactile input. Fine and gross motor skill levels are determined. How a child processes information from many channels and puts it together *(sensory integration)* is also assessed. A standard neurological or psychological examination focusing on brain maturation levels is also performed. This allows us to determine if there has been any permanent damage or if one side of the body is functioning differently from the other. This also enables us to determine which area of the brain and, consequently, which areas of functioning are affected. These tests are used to screen for possible problems and as a guide for more comprehensive testing. A brief physical examination also allows us to determine if there are signs of known disorders which affect the brain and also cause seizures. These include spots on the skin, certain facial features, and other abnormalities which have known associations with disorders.

As a last step, blood tests, x-rays, or scans may be ordered to assist in a diagnosis. Not all children need these procedures to establish a diagnosis. However, it should also be pointed out that while this testing helps establish a diagnosis, it does not in any way alter your child's condition or change treatment recommendations which have been made. It may, however, alter the prognosis – particularly in cases where extensive structural damage is found.

Another important part of the diagnostic picture is obtaining information from your child's teacher. Reading reports and records assist in determining what is already being done for her and how she is functioning in her school setting. Educational and psychological test results should be reviewed.From all of the above information a diagnosis is made and a treatment program drawn up.If a child has significant behavior problems, has poor self-esteem, or if there are family problems, a referral to a mental health professional is in order. Maintaining good feelings and family dynamics are essential to the success of a child with epilepsy. Behavior management and modification programs also assist in this area. If a child is hyperactive or easily distracted, proper classroom placement, behavior management techniques, informed parenting, and medication are all intervention strategies that are part of a complete treatment program.

Developmental Problems And Treatments

The goal of the assessment is to pinpoint the exact type of developmental problems your child has. This leads directly to the treatment plan. The following is a general summary of the usual treatments for developmental problems:

Speech and language delays respond to sessions with a speech/language pathologist. If delays are mild to moderate, a child should be seen individually once or twice a week. For more severe language delays, a child may need to be seen three to five times a week. In some sessions, he is alone with the therapist and in other sessions, he is in a small group with other children. In some cases of severe delay, the child may need to be placed in a small class where the teacher is a speech pathologist or in a program which places heavy emphasis on language skills and concepts, with additional individual language sessions.

Fine motor delays and perceptual and sensory integration problems are treated by exercises provided by an occupational therapist. For mild to moderate delays, one to two sessions per week are sufficient. If a child also has muscle tone problems, an additional two to three sessions per week may be needed to improve and maintain improvement. Rarely does a child need more sessions than that. I can think of only a few extreme cases of severe sensory integration problems where I felt occupational therapy was necessary five times per week with techniques used frequently throughout the day.

Gross motor delays and/or muscle tone problems are usually addressed by a physical therapist in sessions held once or twice a week. Pediatric occupational therapists also address these areas. If a child has mild gross motor problems or has skills which are qualitatively poor, special physical education programs may be sufficient to meet his needs and physical or occupational therapy may not be required.

Recommendations for other special programs may also be made. These include resource programs for support by a special education teacher from one to three hours per day. Self contained (special class) programs for children that have learning disabilities or mental retardation are also necessary in some cases. The type of educational input depends on the child's level of functioning on educational and psychological tests. If a child remains in a regular education class, certain adaptations may need to be made to allow information to be presented to him in a more advantageous manner.

So far we have covered the general areas you need to be aware of in having your child assessed. However, there are also certain considerations that have to do with the age of the child being assessed. Very young children need some special assessments and methods of getting those assessments that do not apply to older children. School age children also have some areas unique to their age group. In the next sections, we will cover these special assessments for both sets of children.

Assessing The Development Of Children Under Five

There are several standard infant scales used by professionals to assess the developmental levels of very young children. Intelligence cannot be accurately determined at this age, but you can determine the rate of progress. Delays at this time have been shown to correlate with later retardation, particularly if they are moderate or severe. Rate of progress should be measured at three to six month intervals using the same test at each session for the first three years. This follow-up is important to ascertain if treatment is affecting change and to determine any critical shortcomings.

You will need to look at the skills your child possesses and at whether she is behind, has lost skills, or is not gaining them at the rate she should. It is important that the same test be used again in three to six month intervals to determine her rate of progress, because each test measures specific areas and has been validated for particular groups of special needs children. Again, your child's intelligence is not being determined during these early years, rather, her rate of progress and developmental level are being determined. You will be told a *corrected age*, a *cognitive level*, or a *developmental level*. This will give you a true picture of your child.

For instance, a child who is eighteen months old, but has the speech/language skills of a nine month old, the motor skills of an eight month old, and the cognitive skills of a twelve month old, would have a corrected age of approximately a year. This child is best treated as a one year old, not as an eighteen month old. His toys, games, play, sleep, and emotional needs are not at eighteen months, so it would not be meeting his needs to approach him from that level. He has special needs.

Listed below is a sampling of tests used for this age group to determine developmental levels:

Bayley Scales of Infant Development. These scales assess mental and psychomotor levels, and are used from ages two months to two and a half years. They take about forty-five minutes to administer.

Cattell Infant Intelligence Scale. This scale assesses mental development and intelligence, and is used on ages three months to thirty months. It takes about thirty minutes to administer.

Early Learning Accomplishment Profile (ELAP). This is a simple record of a child's skills using a checklist format. It is used for children ages birth to thirty-six months and takes about fifteen minutes to administer.

BZOCH-LEAGUE Receptive/Expressive Emergent Language Scale (REEL). This scale uses parent reporting to determine a child's level of language skills. It can be used from birth to three years and takes about forty-five minutes to administer.

Houston Test for Language Development. This is a diagnostic assessment of language from which a language age is determined. It is used from birth through age six and takes about thirty minutes per section.

Rockford Infant Developmental Evaluation Scale (RIDES). This test assesses the range of personal/social and self-help skills. Motor and language skills are also measured. It can be used from birth to four years.

Vineland Social Maturity Scale. These scales measure self-help, self-direction, and social relationships. They determine a social age, and can be used from birth to thirty years.

Taking the Test

It is important to make the most of the test situation itself. Schedule the appointment at your child's best time of day. Make sure she is well rested and has had time to warm up to the examiner. The surroundings should be as comfortable and as familiar as possible. Children do better if tested in a familiar environment, ideally in their own homes. If you do have to go out for the testing, and many of us do, bring some favorite toys and food for your child. If you drive to the appointment, make sure you plan to arrive early so that if your child has slept in the car, she will have time to wake up and become alert before the test. If your child is getting sick, or has not fully recovered from being sick, change your appointment.

Observe the actual test if you can, but avoid interfering. Ask before the test begins what role the tester would like you to assume, how much talking you should do during the test, and if you should cue or coach your child. Try to get all this talk over before the test begins to avoid creating unnecessary distractions. After the test is over, make sure you discuss any observed behaviors that were not typical of your child or any skills that she has in other settings. You might be very surprised at your child's performance, and should express all your opinions to the examiner.

You may or may not get the results right after the testing is completed. You will be sent a written report afterward. If you get verbal results, you should also ask for and receive a written report. Don't hesitate to ask when you can expect the report to arrive. Testing should not be an unpleasant experience for you or your child.

When you receive the written report, make sure it is comprehensive. It should be clear enough that someone who has never seen, or might never see, your child has a true picture of her. You may add to the report by writing separately and attaching your comments. Be sure to clearly indicate what information you provided. The report should list what tests were given, how your child performed on each, and exact levels of functioning. The report should also include specific recommendations for services and amount of time for each service. For instance, if physical therapy is recommended, the report should state that two hours of physical therapy are required each week to improve trunk rotation and thereby improve gross motor development. The report should also identify your 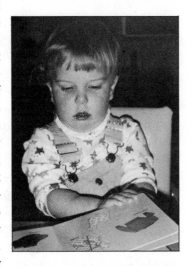 child's learning style. Ideally, we are not just looking at levels of functioning, but also at how a child processes and reacts to stimulation and learns from her environment. Your child's environment and how she responds to it are critical in the approach to meeting special needs. What do things like decoration of the room, light, noise, movement, temperature, and other environmental distractions do to your child? This picture of your child, determined by the evaluation process, will pinpoint what special needs your child has and what specific therapies and educational interventions your child should receive. It will also determine the best educational environment for her optimal participation and learning.

There are steps you can take if you disagree with evaluations of your child. Remember, you are the advocate, the voice for your child. Today, more and more parents are coming to realize that their voice is critical to their child's special education needs. That is not to say that if you do not become involved, your child will receive inferior programs, but to ensure that your child receives the program that is the most appropriate for her as early as possible, you must be actively involved.

The area of assessment and evaluation is the subject of many books, which are listed in the Reading List at the end of this book. I recommend you read as many as you can.

Assessing The Development Of School Age Children

If your child has made it past the infancy stage and met most if not all of the developmental milestones, and can walk and talk, either is, or is on the way to being, potty trained, congratulations! Unless your child develops one of the syndromes associated with intellectual deterioration and motor regression, the development gained during the first two years will, in most cases, not be lost. If your child does regress, essentially the same approach of intense therapy and educational intervention as appropriate for infants is best.

It can be a shattering experience to watch your perfectly normal child regress. You should allow all your feelings to surface during the initial period of acceptance. Just keep in mind that you cannot deny reality nor can you ignore special needs. They must be treated.

In this age group, as in the preschool years, immediate assessment, diagnosis, and treatment is critical. Very often one of the first signs of possible epilepsy is learning problems. Since these problems show up in the classroom, it is the teacher who plays one of the biggest roles in identification, notification, and referral of children who develop seizures. Teachers not only must be keenly aware of the signs of epilepsy and related behavioral effects, but must also be familiar with the range of developmental levels in their classroom. In the end, the teacher is often the one to inform the parents. Hopefully, before that task is performed, the teacher will become aware of community and school referral sources so that the parents can walk away with more than bad news.

In most cases the preschool or regular school has taken a part in the process of identifying your child's special needs through its own screening. Screening is a process used to look at the developmental levels of many children at once and identify children with special needs. This process does not require a highly trained diagnostician and the results usually aid the system in its efforts to identify children who need further assessment.

There are several commonly used screening tests:

Denver Development Screening Test tests for gross motor skills, language skills, fine motor skills, and personal/self-help skills. It can be used for ages six weeks to six years.

The Developmental Indicators for the Assessment of Learning (DIAL) is used to assess children two and a half to five and a half years old. It determines if a child is at risk for learning disabilities, mental retardation, language delay, or speech impairments.

The Pupil Rating Scale: Screening for Learning Disabilities (PRS) tests for learning disabilities. It also checks for the aforementioned skills, however it includes an assessment of orientation (time, special relationships, directions).

As mentioned earlier, there are literally hundreds of developmental tests. The tests mentioned in this text are for informational purposes only and to introduce you to the concept that there are tests to verify any behavioral, cognitive, motor, or social problems you think your child is developing. Don't wait. Early detection is the key to maximizing your child's learning experience.

Once you receive notice that your child needs further evaluation, you again have more choices to make. You can have the evaluation performed by the school system or you can have the testing done privately. It is important for you to decide if your child's needs warrant action that is virtually impossible within some bureaucratic frameworks. Arriving at an accurate diagnosis, treatment plan, appropriate educational placement, and monitoring suitability of this program are the desired outcomes regardless of which sector provides evaluation and assessment. Remember, you and your child should be part of the determining process, part of the team.

How Seizures and Seizure Medications Affect Development and Learning

Seizures and seizure medications can significantly affect development and learning. Frequent seizures reduce your child's ability to process information and respond by disrupting her attention. This disruption occurs not only during overt seizures, but also during subclinical seizure discharges. With tonic/clonic seizures there may be prolonged periods of alterations of the conscious state during and after seizures. The degree to which seizures are controlled directly influences the amount and kind of developmental progress your child makes.

Seizure medication can also affect your child's functioning. Sedation, irritability, and hyperactivity are all negative side effects which affect developmental progress. Phenobarbital has been implicated in the reduction of learning ability, as well as in producing hyperactivity, short attention span, and distractibility.

Learning Problems

Every child is different, but certain patterns which affect learning have been identified as more prevalent among children with epilepsy. These include perceptual/motor problems, delayed verbal skills, and deficits in memory and attention. Studies also show a correlation between certain seizure types—and the area of the brain affected—and particular learning problems. For example, seizures occurring in the right temporal lobe of the brain are linked with certain sensory problems. Lower IQ scores are also found more frequently in children with earlier onset of seizures or a combination of complex partial and generalized seizures.

Many children with epilepsy do not do well in school. Unrecognized or subclinical seizures can be the cause of poor school achievement. The seizures or medication used to treat them can also affect the child's functioning. Difficulties in concentration and memory compound the problem. Studies show that despite normal intelligence thirty-three to seventy percent of children with epilepsy experience learning or school problems. Personality changes, poor motor functioning, and difficulty with reading have been frequently noted.

My advice is to closely monitor your child's school performance for learning problems and to have frequent discussions with your neurologist about suspected problems.

Behavior Problems

Frequently, seizure disorders and other developmental disabilities are accompanied by behavior problems. The most frequently observed behaviors are irritability, temper outbursts, hyperactivity, and attention deficit disorder.

Behavior problems may have been present before any seizures appeared. They can also be complications of the treatment regimen or side effects of antiepileptic drugs. It is important that you try to sort out which of the above phenomena you are actually observing in order to approach the behavior properly. Is the temper outburst caused by frustration? Is it natural temperament? A learned behavior? A seizure phenomenon? Medication will help the latter. Appropriate expectations will alleviate frustrations and a structured behavior program will help eliminate both temperamental and learned behaviors. Hyperactivity and attention deficits can be treated with medication if they are primary disorders, or diminished with a change of medication if they are the side effects of antiepileptic drugs.

In any case, be sure you address your child's behaviors and not just her seizure disorder. Don't presume behaviors are seizure related and will be "cured" by an antiepileptic drug.

Conclusion

Epilepsy can be controlled, but it does not always go away. Epilepsy for many families is disabling, causes handicaps, and creates a whole realm of new needs and services. Your most important role will be that of an informed advocate for your child. Remember, it is up to you. Terms will be unfamiliar or misunderstood. Read. Ask questions, ask for clarifications and examples. Ask again if you feel you have not been given a direct or thorough response. Talk with other parents. Make sure you understand your legal rights. Make sure you participate in all decisions concerning your child.

By working together, we all hope to help children be successful in managing their own conditions. It is my opinion that a child should be given information about his disorder and how it affects him and his world (at home and at school) between the ages of seven to ten. A child should take over control of his medications at age thirteen. He needs to be his own advocate and negotiate to his advantage at school or in society. Knowing his own strengths and weaknesses will allow him to make appropriate choices and avoid frustration. Adolescents will need to discuss their disorders with new emphasis and focus even if this has been done previously. We often forget the child in the process of education and intervention. He is the one who must deal with his handicaps. We will not always be there, nor should we be.

Hopefully, armed with knowledge and your love, your child will be stronger and better able to meet life's challenges than someone who has not been given this opportunity for growth and self-knowledge.

References

Bagley, C.R. "The Educational Performance of Children with Epilepsy." *British Journal of Educational Psychology* 40 (1970): 82–93.

Bourgeois, B.F.D. et al. "Intelligence in Epilepsy: A Prospective Study in Children." *Annals of Neurology* 14 (1983): 438–44.

Cornfield, C.S. et al. "Side Effects of Phenobarbital in Toddlers: Behavioral and Cognitive Aspects." *Journal of Pediatrics* 95 (1979): 361–65.

Dikmen, S. et al. "The Effect of Early Versus Late Onset of Major Motor Epilepsy Upon Cognitive-Intellectual Performance." *Epilepsia* 16 (1975): 73–81.

Guardani, B. et al. "Intelligence Test Performance of Patients with Partial and Generalized Seizures." *Epilepsia* 26 (1985): 37–42.

Keith, H.M. et al. "Mental Status of Children with Convulsive Disorder." *Neurology* 5 (1955): 419–25.

Millichap, J.G. *The Hyperactive Child with Minimal Brain Dysfunction*. Chicago: Year Book Medical Publishers, 1975.

Quinn, P.O. and J.L. Rappaport. "Minor Physical Anomalies and Neurologic Status in Hyperactive Boys." *Pediatrics* 53 (1974): 742–47.

Parent Statements

Stephen was in the middle of eighth grade. His grades dropped drastically. We thought it was a typical teenage rebellion. He was spacy and difficult to handle. He was especially angry. The doctor immediately told us that he was probably using drugs, that it was a phase, and to stick with him through it.

═══✤═══

Even though I knew there's a proper way of dressing her and feeding her, and that I should exercise her daily, I wasn't going to do it. I knew myself well enough to say, "I'm not doing this. I want a break, I want to get away. I can't confront the problem now." But somebody's got to do it. That's why I hired supplemental. It was psychological help for me as well as physical help for Dana.

She's cute, but the older she gets, the more obvious it becomes. She doesn't walk and she doesn't talk. She's four now. She has no receptive language, although she does respond to tone. The older she gets the more questions I see in peoples' eyes.

Endless baby! When is the baby going to grow up, when is the crying going to end, when is she going to stop wearing a diaper?

I finally realized that I allow him to feed himself, make a mess, run the cream of wheat through his hair only when I'm in the mood, when I'm relaxed and can deal with the mess. When I'm not in the mood, I take the spoon and feed him. I give him a toy to play with so I don't have to deal with it.

The thing I'm about to do is set up a group in case management to help people round out their worlds. I've found that there are so many splinter groups. You can go through the medical field and they know their medical people. You can go through the education field and they know their people. I haven't found anyone who's case managing it and helping direct people. Why should it be such a lonely vigil for parents to go through these step-by-step procedures without any help?

I never ever would have guessed that raising a child with a disability, even a minor one, would be such an enormous expense.

When we took Kirsten to be evaluated for her developmental disabilities one of the first things we were told by the evaluator was to move to another county where the services will meet her needs; where you can get the best your tax dollar will provide.

Because our first child developed seizures at such a young age we never experienced normal development. When our second came along, we were, and continue to be, amazed at normal development.

We have occupational, physical, and speech therapists. He's in a special school; we've seen a developmental pediatrician, hearing specialists, a pediatric epileptologist, a family psychologist, and miscellaneous specialists as we're referred to them. We didn't know there were so many different professionals to deal with one kid. It's a job to keep it coordinated.

He might have trouble opening a jar. It's not because he forgot how to do it, it's because he doesn't have the control over his muscles. As far as his intelligence—he knows and can do everything he once could—new learning is slow but it's still there.

He's always been somewhat delayed but we thought he'd mature eventually. He didn't walk until he was eighteen months. He didn't really talk until three years.

I know that there are many children that live normal lives and still have epilepsy. Sometimes I resent how developmentally delayed our daughter is. Epilepsy has such a broad range of problems associated with it.

I think when you see Henry and talk with him you know there's something that's not entirely right but you really can't identify it. As soon as professionals are told he has epilepsy, they automatically treat him different-ly. They overreact to all his behavior. They over-do it.

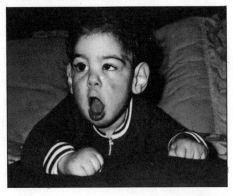

At one year old, he can-not sit up or hold his head up. He cannot hold a toy in his hand. He cannot roll over. He has very little head control. The seizures make it impossible for him to learn; developmentally, his corrected age is one month. He is very hard to feed; each meal takes about one hour.

The seizures began to abate and stopped about six months ago. Miraculously Robbie started to learn and say things, to do the small tasks that are major victories for kids like ours. He is now toilet trained which is as close to Nirvana as we have approached.

There is no professional who looks at the child as a whole person. Each one looks at certain parts of his or her body. Parents are often confused.

Since Ray's diagnosis, we have been inundated with a vocabulary of terms we'd never even heard of. There's so much new information for us to learn so we can discuss his problems with the professionals.

I guess it could be a crutch, an excuse, a way out, to blame poor performance on drugs or epilepsy. But how on earth can we ever know if the seizures or medicine side effects are the cause? What is our base line?

His epilepsy has given us more anxious hours and threatened his life more than anything. His deafness, cortical blindness, curvature of the spine, and Cerebral Palsy needed attention, but his epilepsy was nerve-racking. It required constant vigilance.

He has a lot of equipment to safeguard him. He has headgear, a seat belt, padded tray, and head rest on his wheelchair. He sleeps in an adult sized crib. He can't stand but can get to an upright kneeling position and therefore a bed with hospital side rails would not guard him from somersaulting over the side during a seizure.

Epilepsy was just a minor facet of his overall condition. But the management of his epilepsy was a major stress, financial burden, and took an enormous amount of family time.

I wish we could get a straight answer on Ray's progress and what it means as far as retardation goes. I've never encountered beating around the bush the way I have when I bring up the word "retardation." It's unbelievable.

Our son has been evaluated, assessed, tested, rated, and charted so many times during these past two years that we've lost count. We still don't know much about him. He's different after every seizure.

When the team sits down with us and shares their evaluation results, I am stunned. In a state of shock. I can't believe what I'm hearing. Epilepsy has really screwed up our little girl. Will the special education and therapy really help?

I can see how easy it would be to take for granted the normal, effortless development that most children experience. Everything Ray does is like a miracle to us.

Facing the reality of having a child with special needs takes a lot of guts, a lot of painful adjustment, and a lot of personal growth. But once you do what you have to do and move on, keep on moving and don't get stuck in a stage. Then life is okay again. There is happiness in watching your special little child develop.

SEVEN

An Introduction To Special Education

LINDA DIAMOND, M.S.; SHARON ANDERSON, O.T.R., NDT
CERTIFIED; HELENE BERK, M.ED.; AND ROMAYNE SMITH,
M.A., CCC-SP.*

Many children with epilepsy do not suffer developmental delays or disabilities. Unfortunately, some children do. If you have just learned that your child needs special education, you may be feeling overwhelmed and unequipped to find services. This chapter will help you become familiar with the range of services usually found in special education programs and will also discuss the relationship between parents and special education professionals. As with neurology, special education has a language all its own. Please refer to the Glossary at the back of this book.

Thanks to parents and advocates, Public Law 94–142 makes sure that our educational system works to help our children learn, regardless of their disability. (See chapter 8 for more details.) Special Education is education designed for your child, based on an Individualized Educational Plan (IEP) *which is carefully designed for your child's precise needs*. You are a part of the program planning and monitoring. You are

---

* The authors make up a transdisciplinary team at the Ivymount School in Rockville, Maryland. Linda Diamond is the Family Coordinator, Sharon Anderson is the Occupational & Physical Therapy Coordinator, Helene Berk is a Special Education teacher, and Romayne Smith is a Speech/Language Pathologist.

a member of the team. The law provides that whenever possible our children do not have to be isolated in special schools, but mainstreamed into regular classes and with children in regular educational placements.

Since you are part of the team identifying your child's educational needs, you need to learn about special education. Then you can work hand in hand with the school professionals to help your child reach his optimal level of functioning.

What Is Special Education?

Special education means specially designed instruction to meet the unique needs of the handicapped child. It can take place in the classroom, and when necessary in the home or a hospital. In addition, special education can include what are called "related services" like physical and occupational therapy, speech therapy, psychological and social services, and transportation.

Professionals

The special education services discussed above are provided by a wide variety of professionals, usually referred to as a multidisciplinary team. Although titles and specific areas of responsibility can differ from place to place, the following is a review of the special education professionals you may encounter:

Special Education Teacher. A special education teacher is trained in using specific techniques for teaching children who have difficulty learning in the regular educational setting. She will look closely at your child's overall development and particularly at cognitive development.

Physical Therapist. A physical therapist works with your child on the sequential development of motor skills. Special attention is given to developing the quality of movement patterns and to increasing strength and endurance.

Occupational Therapist. An occupational therapist works with your child on a variety of sensory motor skills, including: 1) receiving and using sensory input for accurate movement and organization of behavior, 2) using the small muscles of the face, eye, and hands for skilled functions, and 3) using large and small muscles in combination to perform activities in daily life like eating, dressing, and toileting.

Speech and Language Therapist (Pathologist). This therapist is often referred to as a speech therapist and works with your child's communication skills. Both receptive and expressive language, as well as development of articulation of sounds and words, is included. Oral sensory and oral motor development (use of the muscles in and around the mouth) are also evaluated.

Mental Health Professional. Some special education programs have counselors, social workers, family coordinators, and mental health professionals available to help children and parents cope with epilepsy and its effects.

Programs

The professionals mentioned above work in many different kinds of settings. Special education programs differ from place to place, and it is important for you to learn about the types of programs available to your child. These are some general guidelines to the different types of programs.

Family Centered vs. Child Centered. Some programs focus on just the child in special education and are termed "child centered." Their philosophy is that services should be provided to the child himself. These types of programs do not offer services to the parents or families. Other 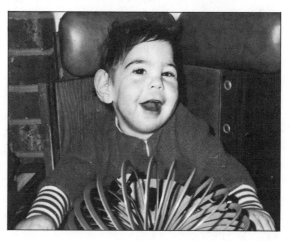 programs are "family centered." They focus on both the child and the family, looking at how best to integrate the special needs child into the family.

Center Based vs Home Based. Educational services are usually provided in a school center or at home. In a center based program the child goes to school and is brought to a classroom, sometimes called activity or resource room, for work with other children with similar needs. In home based services, the special education team comes to your home. This type of program is offered when a child's health is fragile or at risk.

Planning Your Child's Educational Program

You will be working closely with a special education teacher. She will look at the following areas as she plans how best to teach him.

Skill Levels

- Cognitive, thinking/problem solving;
- Pre-academic or academic skills;
- Social-emotional development, including self-esteem, peer interactions, and work habits;
- Overall developmental levels, including gross and fine motor, language, and self-help. A delay in a particular skill area can affect your child's performancein another area. For example, a child with delayed fine motor skills might have difficulty holding a pencil to write efficiently.

Strengths and Weaknesses

A child might have strong visual motor skills and poor receptive language skills. In other words, the child might be able to look and figure out how to do something, but can't understand the same thing if he had to listen to directions. The teacher can use this information to plan lessons that use his strengths. By not just relying on the child's comprehension of language, the teacher can help improve his chances of learning.

Attention Span and Interest

Can your child work on an activity for one minute, five minutes, or thirty minutes? Will he work better if the school day is frequently broken up with motor/movement activities? What things interest and motivate him? Does he work better in a quiet environment? Is he distracted by classmates or when working in a group?

Developmental Patterns

Does it take a long time to learn new skills or does he learn quickly? Does he practice a newly learned task repeatedly before he tries the next one or does he "spurt" and learn a number of new skills together? Does he "plateau" regularly?

Adaptive behavior

How has he made adjustments in his skills to function in his environment? Can he generalize skills from one situation to another? Does he use learned skills in everyday functioning? How a child uses known skills is an important consideration when determining cognitive functioning. Observers such as teachers, caregivers, and parents can provide extremely important input about adaptive behavior.

By looking at your child's strengths and weaknesses, attention span, interests, and developmental patterns, the teacher determines your child's learning style. This information, along with your child's skill levels, will be used as a basis to set up a classroom environment to meet *your child's special needs*. Note that we emphasize plans and programs to meet your child's unique educational needs. This is the essence of special education.

Placing Your Child in a Program

The information gathered about your child will be used to help determine the most appropriate placement. Children who are just entering a program will probably have an initial assessment done by the school. As discussed in Chapter 6, testing done by a developmental pediatrician or clinic may also be used in determining placement. If your child is already in a program, information from professionals and parents about the previous school year is also helpful in determining placement. It is a good idea to keep in mind that if necessary a placement can change at any time during the school year.

Placements can differ in many way, according to your child's needs.

Level of Service. This is the amount of special education your child needs. It can vary from a full day in a special education class to remaining in a regular class with a special education/resource teacher 30 minutes a day who gives help in one particular area.

Model of Program. Variations can include the size of the classroom, staff/student ratios, structured or less structured programs, level of family involvement, and an emphasis on an academic program or functional living program.

Talk to professionals, advocacy organizations, and other parents in your community about specific program options available for your child. Read the recommended books in the Reading List about special education.

Integrating Your Child in the Classroom

Once your child has been placed in a classroom, the special education teacher will do the following:

1. Get to know your child through observations through formal and informal evaluations. A teacher might use both standardized tests and teacher checklists. School curriculums are designed so children must master certain skills at one academic level before moving on to the next because those skills are necessary for success at the next level. Your child's teacher is the best source for information on your child's individual skill assessment.

2. After obtaining information on individual children, your child's teacher will look at the overall make up of the class.

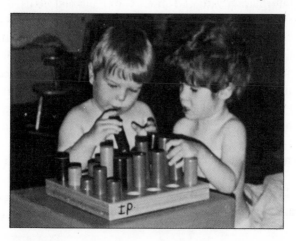

She will consider things like who might work well together and who might tire easily. She will then plan the overall schedule, and each individual child's classroom day with the above information in mind. For example: How long should activities last? How often should table activities be alternated with movement and less structured activities?

3. Coordinate with other professionals working with your child. These might include a physical therapist, an occupational therapist, a speech/language therapist, a pediatrician, and a neurologist. Your teacher will want to know about your child's seizures and medications. Sharing all this information will help her plan the best education program for your child.

4. Share her observations and evaluations with you. In order to plan the best program for your child, she will need to confirm her observations or hear differences seen at home or in other settings (babysitter, previous school.)

5. Use information to develop an IEP with you and other members of the team. There are many resources and books listed in the Reading List at the back of this book if you want to learn more about the IEP. The school is responsible, by law, to provide all the instruction that is on the IEP, including related services, such as physical therapy. The IEP should list the area of instruction, the current level of performance, and the annual goal, and then identify short-term objectives leading to the annual goal. Remember, the IEP is an *individualized* education program and no two are alike. It is designed for your child's individual needs.

6. Plan lessons for your child that carry through his IEP goals and objectives.

7. Monitor your child's progress. This might be through teacher checklists, observations, and periodic informal and formal tests. Many teachers develop ongoing communication with parents to share school progress, as well as receive information about home. It may be through a notebook, home visits, or phone calls. If your child's teacher does not have this set up, you should do it. Your role as a member of the team is to provide monitoring and your input is critical. For example, your child may be doing things at home that he is not doing

at school. Your child's teacher should know about this progress.

Occupational And Physical Therapy

As your child enters the world of special education, two important professionals that may be a part of your child's team are the occupational therapist (OT) and the physical therapist (PT). Depending on the extent and area of your child's needs, he may have both or only one of these therapists as a part of his educational team. Both of these therapists are described earlier.

Because the areas of occupational and physical therapy are so interrelated, it is easy to see similarities in treatment activities. A good example would be seen in the treatment goal of establishing improved trunk control. The physical therapist must work toward this goal as a prerequisite to sitting and walking; the occupational therapist works toward the same goal as a prerequisite to sitting and using the arms for feeding or other skilled activities.

The first thing an occupational therapist or physical therapist will do with your child is begin assessing your child's skills and problems, looking not only at what he can do but also at the quality of the movements. This assessment process will probably be both formal and informal. Informal assessment may consist of parent interviews and ongoing observation; formal assessment may consist of giving gross and fine motor development tests, tests of sensory integration, tests of visual motor (eye/hand coordination) control, and tests of visual perception.

Assessing Your Child's Sensory Motor Development

The occupational therapist and/or physical therapist will evaluate the following areas before beginning a treatment plan.

Gross Motor. Reflex maturation, muscle tone, range of motion, righting and equilibrium reactions, transitional movements (from one position to another), motor milestones, quality of movement and quantity of movement. In other words, how well does your child use his body?

Fine Motor. Proximal control, isolation of movement, grasp and release, in-hand manipulation, ocular motor control, visual perception, handedness, and tool use. In other words, how well does your child do thing like put together puzzles, draw and reach for things. **Sensory Organization.** Initial response and adaptation to: visual input, sound, touch, movement, and gravity, position, taste, and smell, and self regulatory behaviors (ability to calm, organize behavior, maintain attention). In other words, how does your child receive all the messages from his basic senses and what does he do with them. **Self Help.** Feeding, dressing, toileting, grooming.

Occupational and physical therapists usually determine your child's level of development and work on treatment goals that are pertinent to educational development. The first aim of treatment is to provide basic building blocks so that more normal development can occur. These important building blocks are a balanced sensory system and normal movement. For example a child who cannot tolerate touch, usually referred to as tactile defensive would not be able to tolerate being handled in a treatment session or be able to use his hands very well until his tactile system is in better balance. The next aim would be to work on refinement of skills so that the child could become more independent. For example, with a child who is just beginning to shift weight from one foot to the other, the next goal would be using both feet to climb up and down steps. In some cases a child's development may be so impaired that changes do not occur. If this is the case, a therapist will look at what skills would enhance the child's quality of life and find other strategies and equipment. An example of this would be the child who did not have the physical ability to become an independent walker. The therapist could then help in the fitting, ordering, and training for an electric wheelchair.

As you read about the services that occupational and physical therapists provide, you may wonder how these therapies fit into the special education setting and how the service will be delivered. Public Law 94–142 identifies occupational and physical therapy as a related service. This means the therapy must be provided if it is necessary to help your child learn.

Direct occupational and physical therapy are provided in many schools by therapists who are employed by the school. Other school systems contract for therapy services from public health departments, hospitals, and private occupational and physical therapy practices.

If your child is very young, occupational and physical therapy services may be provided in your home. With young children, it is best to have the therapist on the team available not only for direct treatment, but also for ongoing consultation with other team members, including you.

As your child becomes older, there are different models of treatment. The most common form is individual treatment in a specially designed treatment room. Other models range from individual treatment to small groups. In most cases, the optimal is a combination of in class and individual treatment. If the therapist can be in the class instructing other staff on how to assist your child to move, and to hold a pencil, for example, he will benefit greatly.

Occupational and physical therapists have extensive clinical training experience before certification. Many physical and occupational therapists have specialized training in Neurodevelopmental Treatment (NDT). NDT stands for neurodevelopment treatment which is a form of therapy used on people who have central nervous system disorders resulting in abnormal movement. The name comes from the words "neuro" for brain and nerves, and "development" for growth and maturation.

An additional certification therapists might have is sensory integration certification . This is commonly called SI. Sensory integration is the ability to organize the messages sent by the brain. These sensations include what we see, hear, taste, and smell, and also what we feel from the pull of gravity, from moving around, and from all our muscle, bone, and skin receptors. A child with good sensory integration has a nervous system that is able to sort and direct sensations into a smooth flow, rather like a traffic cop. The child can use this integrated information to form concepts, develop relationships, and otherwise adapt to his environment. The system of a child with poor sensory interaction is not able to direct sensory motor traffic in any organized fashion. His sensory integration could be described as a traffic jam. Occupational and physical therapists trained in sensory integration can help the child with problems in this area.

Teaching Language To Your Child

A speech and language therapist is often one of the special education team members for important reasons. First, communication is such a critical area: much of the rest of learning depends upon it. Second, communication is part of functioning in our world. Third, the development of language and speech skills also depends on cognitive, motor, social, and emotional development.

Seizures and speech/language impairment may be related. The underlying neurological problem that may have led to the seizure disorder could have also disrupted the normal development or functioning of the speech and language areas of the brain. The seizures themselves may cause a child to be unable to take in and process language.

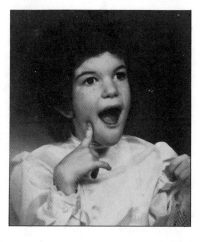

Perhaps your child is young enough so that he is just beginning to learn language. Your child's speech therapist will point out to you the way you naturally stimulate language and speech skills. She will provide guidelines for ways you can do this with more awareness. The therapist will ask you to use language at your child's level of understanding. Often children with developmental delays understand more than they can express. This means you will need to talk to stimulate expressive and receptive levels of language.

Often audiologists (hearing specialists) are not found on special education teams. As a result, the speech therapist will want to obtain information about your child's hearing and determine whether any middle ear problem exists. A hearing problem could interfere with your child's communication. This information will come from an independent hearing evaluation.

For some children with speech and language delays, the speech therapist and the special education teacher may feel that spoken language should be augmented with other communication methods. The methods most often used with young children are gestures and signs (taken from sign systems used by hearing impaired people), and communication or picture boards/books. Giving some children additional visual cues can help them make sense of what they are hearing and help them learn to speak themselves. This last point is critical: both clinical experience and research show that augmentative language systems do not deter—but rather—increase the likelihood that children will speak. Many children combine systems by talking while they sign or use pictures to communicate. Often, augmentative systems will be a temporary step in your child's development.

Communication requires skill and practice. Language is used to both express and to respond. Long before they begin to talk, infants learn how to take turns in a conversation and how to keep dialogue going between themselves and others. For example, does your child call out to get your attention or acknowledge he has heard when you call him? Does he have a question to ask? Does he want to comment on something of interest to him?

If your child's neurological development is disrupted at an early age, his communication skills may not develop normally. In the last few years speech therapists and special educators have become aware that some children with developmental disabilities do not learn on their own. These children do not seem to realize the possibility for reaching out and initiating interactions, but wait passively for an adult to make the first overture.

Another important area your child's speech therapist will monitor is syntax and grammar. Syntax or grammar is the collection of rules for combining words to express yourself. When speech/language therapists use the term grammar, they do not mean "proper English," but rather the way in which people ordinarily talk. There is a regular developmental sequence children go through as they begin to combine two and three words. Therapists also look at the way words are changed to make their meanings more distinct. For example, fly becomes flies; the order by which it joins other words changes its meaning: "I hate flies" or "She flies faster." The speech therapist will check to see whether your child has the grammatical rules expected for his language and cognitive age.

Another area of intervention for a child with delayed speech is work on the sensory and motor skills of his face, head, and mouth; perhaps even the rest of his body. This kind of approach to helping speech along may be carried out by a speech or occupational therapist. The goal is to help your child develop skill moving his jaw, tongue, and lips to make speech sounds, and control the air stream required to make those sounds. Infants and very young children may need work on developing oral skills for eating and drinking.

Your child may need therapy outside school. The least may be that he is monitored periodically. If more is necessary the therapist will compare what your child understands to his cognitive level to determine whether they match. She will then develop a speech therapy plan to help his talking match what he understands.

The therapist will also look at how delayed a skill area is in relation to others. The milder the problem, the less time she will recommend that your child spend in therapy each week. Another factor to consider is how much structured language therapy the child is receiving from the teacher.

If your baby is not using some basic skills, such as eye contact, turn-taking in conversation, and using noises to initiate interactions, beyond the ages of three to six months, it is recommended that you get a speech and language evaluation. Language skills are developing most rapidly at these earlier ages.

If your child did not develop epilepsy until elementary school age or older, his speech may not have been affected very much. Perhaps the only effect is missed information or understanding during the actual seizure itself, or just afterward. Have his speech evaluated and start therapy if necessary.

Getting Started

As mentioned in the previous chapter, there may be a doctor, teacher, or counselor who you trust who would be able to help you as you learn what to do and when. Also, the EFA (Epilepsy Foundation of America) or other groups, such as ACLD (Association for Children with Learning Disabilities), ARC (Association for Retarded Citizens), and many others may have chapters in your area. They can provide you with information about special education services and provide tips on how to negotiate the process. The books in the Reading List at the back of this book are highly recommended resources. A parent who has already negotiated the special education maze is also an invaluable resource.

Remember, you know your child, you are the expert on your child and family. You will be coming in contact with many people in your local school system as you find out what special services are offered and how they match what has been recommended for your child. Step back for a moment and make sure you understand the information that has been given to you. Do you understand how your child's strengths and needs are viewed? Do you agree? Do you have a clear understanding of what services have been recommended and why? If you are unclear about any of this information, get a clear explanation before you start working with the school system since, at least initially, you will have to be teaching the educators about your child.

Becoming Part Of The Team

Every school system is unique, although certain services are mandated by the law. It is important that you are able to communicate the information about your child accurately, and to have a sense of whether the services offered can meet your child's needs. You are a part of the decision-making team. Some school systems encourage this participation and others do not. But, regardless of their approach, you have the right and responsibility to ask questions, request information, observe programs that are being considered, and be an active part of the decision-making process. It is well worth the effort to try to communicate with professionals and to ultimately form a team with them. This involves getting information about decisions made for and about your child and not relying solely on the professionals to do this.

Depending on the needs of your child, you will encounter a variety of programs and at least one of the professionals described in this chapter. Also, depending again on your child's age and needs and the individual program there will be differing degrees of involvement of the family in planning. Generally, family involvement and daily contact decreases as the child gets older. However, you should expect, and request if necessary, to always be part of the decision-making team with the professionals serving your child.

Optimally, family members will be considered a vital part of the team, beginning with evaluations, moving on to making decisions about the best program, and continuing with service. However, it is your responsibility to make this happen. Ultimately, you will have to be the long-term case manager for your child. Professionals can take this role at times, but they should be helping you gain the knowledge and skills necessary for you to take over. Professionals are your consultants. They have expertise in a variety of fields and will know your child from an educational viewpoint. However, you have the long-term overall knowledge and responsibility. Professionals can help you to feel more competent with your child, but the job is yours.

Some professionals will be open and honest in sharing information and will make every attempt to include your input in decision making. Sometimes, this is not the case. Professionals may seem reticent to share information or become defensive when you ask questions. Many professionals were not trained to work with parents. Sometimes the questions asked may evoke insecure feelings; feelings of needing to be the expert and know all the answers rather than to brainstorm with you; feelings of having to "fix" everything and not knowing how to respond to upset parents. None of these issues are your responsibility and none are things which should concern you. However, they are part of the reality of working with professionals and if you are aware of these issues, then perhaps you will be able to work around them to get the best possible results for you and your child.

In order to establish a parent/professional relationship based on respect and trust, here are some suggestions:

- Be honest and clear in what you are asking for; share your concerns as openly as you can.
- Don't be intimidated; remember, you do know your child. If you feel intimidated, however, try to admit it freely and keep on working.
- Don't expect the professionals to have all the answers, or a magic solution; ask them to brainstorm with you. They are the experts in the field. You are the expert on your child and family. You need to work together to find the answers.
- Ask for the information you need. No question is a stupid one.
- It is okay to disagree and work toward a resolution.

- Share your child's history and your present concerns, expectations, and hopes for the future for your child and family. Remember that you have a great deal of specific information. No one knows your child the way you do.
- Give the professionals time to get to know your child.
- You can expect to be told some initial observations. It is important to work out when you will talk about your child. Find options that will work for all of you. Ask directly and try to have a few options that would be acceptable. For instance, if drop off and pick up times are not workable for the teacher, how about a phone call or a short daytime meeting?

Communication

As your child begins his education, professionals will be asking many questions about behaviors at home. They are getting to know your child. Ask them about his school behavior, then compare the results and discuss your findings with the other members of your team. This can be important from the perspective of learning how your child is adjusting to school, how he relates to other people, and how he uses his skills away from home. This process is the beginning of the give and take of communication necessary to build a partnership between you and the people working with your child.

At times, sharing your concerns or questions may make you feel vulnerable, because you are taking a risk with professionals you may not know or trust. Take some time to develop a relationship, but remember, the more you are able to be open and clear with your communication, the more you will help create the trust and sense of team. Listening openly to what others are saying is crucial to building good communication and working relationships. Try to listen actively to what others are saying. For example, if a teacher says something you do not understand, simply ask, "I think what I heard you say was that Susan will be the youngest one in the class. Exactly what does that mean? Does it only mean that she'll be the youngest, or did you intend to say more?" The professionals should function as consultants to you and have a great deal of important information and a perspective to share with you.

Remember, emotions can often cloud the facts and issues and interfere with clear communication. This happens to both parents and professionals. Try to be aware of when this is happening and let the other person know. You can ask a friend to accompany you, take notes, or tape record meetings. Sometimes, communication will fall apart. If you have a partnership, don't worry, communication will be re-established.

None of this is easy. If the professionals take equal responsibility for creating and maintaining this partnership, it can be very rewarding. If you are fighting the tides, it can be frustrating. However, a partnership is the best arrangement and something worth pursuing.

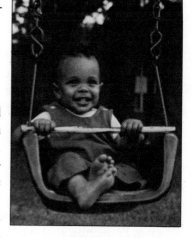

Working With The Family

There will be a professional who will help you as you work with the different members on your team. She might be called the family co-ordinator, social worker, guidance counselor, or psychologist.

Families who have children with special needs are placed in an extraordinary position which creates stress. In addition to the emotional factors involved in having a child with special needs, parents find themselves in need of learning information and advocacy techniques. Therefore, many comprehensive special education programs (family centered) provide families with support services and a specific relationship will be developed to provide that support.

In many programs, there are regularly scheduled parent group meetings. These often focus on exchanging information and support. Many parents find that talking with other parents, hearing similar experiences, and making friends with families in the same boat very comforting. In some programs, siblings may also be offered this individual service as well as a support group.

The person responsible for the family coordination can help you locate resources you may need for services outside your child's program. She can help you learn to advocate for yourself and your child. She often works very closely with people directly serving your child and can be the staff person bringing family issues to team discussions. She can support and guide staff in their efforts to see your child as part of a family as well as guide the team discussion toward meeting family needs.

Depending on your program, you may meet with the family professional when initially setting up your child's individual program. This is a time not only for gathering factual information, but also for beginning the process of educating the staff about your child's needs, your concerns, and your family. It is also the time for you to learn the ins and outs of the program.

The team's overall goal is to help your child learn and develop and to minimize his handicap. Another goal is to share information in order to give you a realistic idea of the impact his handicap will have in the long run. The long-term goal for your family is to be able to help your child, to integrate his special needs into the family, and to function as a family unit.

Case Studies

The following examples illustrate the different ways that special education can help children with learning problems associated with epilepsy. Remember that every child is unique, his epilepsy, although of the same seizure type as another child's, causes unique reactions, different outcomes, and different functioning levels. Epilepsy in and of itself does not create a category or a range of expectations. These case studies are presented just to show how the different types of programs and professionals can work in practice and give you some ideas about what special education program to set up for your child.

Alexander is a ten-year-old boy who had absence seizures diagnosed at age nine and a half. His family and school were unable to say whether or not it had been going on for very long, or suddenly became apparent. His seizures are successfully controlled by medication. Alexander attends regular education, but he has gaps in academic skills and a very poor sense of self-esteem. He displays aggressive acting-out behavior and generally seems frustrated. He receives one hour a week in a resource room for specific help on academic gaps. The special education resource teacher coordinates with the classroom teacher, resulting in a team approach to his needs. A social worker sees him individually and in a peer group situation to foster self-esteem and model appropriate social interactions. His parents also see the social worker periodically to support school goals at home and share their concerns.

Sue is a five year old who developed infantile spasms at three months of age. She was treated with ACTH, which was successful and she is now medication free. Her development in all skill areas proceeded slowly. She showed severe attention deficits and poor impulse control. At two-and-one half years, her development accelerated. At five years she shows delays in her speech and language skills. She finds it difficult to function in a normal kindergarten class since she is unable to focus on her teacher's voice with background voices present. She can understand speech, but to do so, she must concentrate a little more than most children her age. Therefore a smaller, quieter classroom environment is to her educational advantage. She receives this in a special education classroom. She is seen by the speech therapist three times a week at school. An occupational therapist also sees her twice a week for sensory integration therapy and works on her fine motor skills as well as reinforces the speech therapist's goals. She no longer receives physical therapy because the quality and level of her gross motor skills are age appropriate. Family services continue to develop parenting skills to meet her special attention and distractibility problems.

Jason is an eight-month-old boy who developed neonatal seizures. His medication does not control his seizures well. He is beginning to hold his head up. He cannot sit, he dislikes being touched or held, tends to be irritable, and is difficult to calm. He responds to voices and smiles occasionally. He has some difficulty sucking liquids from a bottle and taking food from a spoon. He responds to a toy, but is unable to reach and grasp. His parents experience continual sadness and depression about having a baby who may always be handicapped. Due to very significant delays in all areas of development and serious health problems, Jason is receiving comprehensive integrated special education services. This includes home visits from an infant special educator with occupational and speech therapists working as part of the team providing early intervention. A physical therapist also sees Jason weekly. The family coordinator works with the parents individually and as a couple. She also works with the total family, including the three siblings. The parents participate in a monthly parent support group.

Matthew is a six year old who developed Lennox-Gastaut syndrome at age four. His development up until that time was normal. He experienced severe intellectual regression as well as motor deterioration as a result of the seizures. He also lost all toileting skills and had to go back to diapers. In order to protect his head from the drop attacks, he wore a protective helmet for two years and has just begun going without it. He attends a special education class in a school that is for developmentally delayed and retarded students, up to age twenty-one. His classroom is staffed by a special educator and an aide. He also has an aide assigned solely to him to help him with his fine motor skills, such as holding a pencil, a cup, and various educational tools. The aide also helps train him to relearn his toileting skills as well as help him to regain his other lost skills. He is one of eight children in his classroom, which is air conditioned. He is also provided with an air conditioned taxi cab to drive him to and from school, since none of the school buses in his school district have air conditioning. His parents state that his seizures are much worse during hot and humid weather, therefore the school district provided appropriate transportation. It would have been an inappropriate placement if he had to endure an atmosphere that lowered his seizure threshold. He receives speech, occupational, and physical therapy for one hour apiece each week, and the therapists coordinate with the classroom staff so that he gets consistent language and positioning input.

Conclusion

One of the most important messages from the special education community is that YOU are a part of the team. You are the specialist professionals look to for insight into your child's strengths, weaknesses, learning style, and adaptive behavior. Your experience with your child is crucial to placement decisions, program planning, and monitoring. You have the expertise to plan the IEP along with the team and to make critical decisions about mainstreaming. Never forget, special education is instruction designed specifically for your child's educational needs, based on a comprehensive evaluation of his strengths and weaknesses. The system provides trained specialists and ongoing revision of program goals.

It is also a good idea for the people responsible for our children's care, whether they are parents or professionals, to consider the reality of life after the protection of Public Law 94–142 is over. What will there be for our children after the school years? Ensure a future by including vocational planning in the IEP. Encourage as much self-sufficiency as possible by becoming involved in your child's special education.

You have a difficult job ahead of you, but as we have pointed out in this chapter, there are many people and systems available to help you. With your guidance, your child can get the best possible education available.

Parent Statements

I don't know if this is a false hope that we have, but I keep thinking the more we do for him now – more services, more therapy, stimulation, and everything else, it'll help him reach whatever self-sufficiency he's capable of.

I fought a special education placement for a long time. I really believed that with will power you could do anything you wanted to do – so I kept him in a regular school for four years. I just became convinced recently that he'd be better off in a special program. Next year he'll go to a language impaired disability program.

Some people do a lot of reading. I don't know why but I couldn't read. I tried but I listened the most. I learned so much from the occupational therapist that came here to the house. She taught me almost everything.

You know how the therapists give you little exercises. This is how you're supposed to pick them up, bend the knee this way and the leg dangling this way and everything. After a while it's just pick 'em up, thirty-five pounds is enough already, who cares how you get it up.

He was a straight A student, very, very bright. He was always a pretty shy kid but this has made him withdraw even more. His grades were always a source of pride. Now, no matter how hard he works he only gets C's. He's in a learning resource center.

I just think whatever is wrong with him as far as the seizures go is also causing the developmental problems. He's got real processing problems. The seizures are just one manifestation and the developmental problems another.

It was the school that let me know he was having seizures. They'd notice his eyes flickering, or just stare for a second or so. That really makes learning impossible. I'm so grateful his teachers and I work together on this. Otherwise, I'd never have known.

I was fighting special ed because of old stereotypes from my childhood. "Language impaired" is such a heavy label. Now I realize the enormous benefit for him and how far forward our society and educational system has progressed. I thank God we've got special ed now.

He's in speech therapy every day. Three days by himself and two days with other kids. They play games, do word drills, tell stories; things like that. His school is excellent. It's public.

I was the one who said, "Please put her in both classes. She's not getting anything from the more profoundly handicapped. If you don't present both opportunities, how's she going to learn?" If we need to get an aide for her to be in the more advanced class, then that's what the school district and I will talk about because that's what's within my rights.

I had a very hard time getting them to separate the epilepsy from his learning disability. They'd say he's doing this because of the epilepsy or that because of the epilepsy instead of saying, "It doesn't really matter why all this is going on. What are we going to do about it?" We were stuck in a "why is he doing this?" mode for a year and half.

The most important thing we can do is give job counseling and provide opportunities to learn job skills. Learning hobbies is great fun but they don't usually translate into jobs. After age twenty-one, parents must be fully in charge. There is no support from the outside. All those school years just end, Bam.

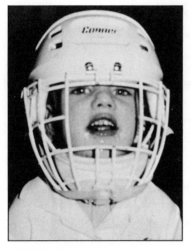

The varied tactile stimulation he desperately needed was denied him because of the constant seizing. The toys on his wheelchair tray were severely limited to a boring variation of crash-safe rattles and rubber duckies.

The teachers have been so helpful, explaining epilepsy to the students and making it seem okay. It's made it easier for his brothers and sisters. They don't feel as ashamed or embarrassed now.

Obviously he's not going to be an intellectual so we'll want to get him into a really good vocational program.

I had to get the school's doctor to watch him in class and then call the neurologist. The neurologist talked openly with the school doctor and then he'd pass on the information to the principal and teacher. It was ridiculous since I'd been saying the same things all along.

I think that as long as I put my foot down, they respond. We have to really make school personnel accountable. But sometimes I feel like the obnoxious parent and dread what I am obligated to do.

Regardless of the money we spend on evaluations and specialists, we end up managing and coordinating all the education, the related services, and the doctors. We make sure everybody knows what everyone else is doing. Sometimes when we're writing out another check for a hundred dollars or so, we feel really frustrated because we didn't learn a thing. It seems like educational and medical professionals alike are afraid to put themselves on the line and really say something.

It's important for parents to realize that they must follow their instincts, change therapists if necessary, and believe in themselves and their understanding of their child.

It is critical to remember that your child is still a little kid who needs to play, to be free, to run around without a special teacher or therapist breathing down his neck.

Mainstreamed special education is the opportunity for all of us to create a world of tolerance and understanding. Children that grow and learn with handicapped children have fewer questions or fears about handicaps. Mainstreaming provides the opportunity for children with seizures to become their own advocates and set their own examples to the world. Ultimately, they can become in control of their own lives.

EIGHT

Legal Rights And Hurdles

BY JAMES E. KAPLAN AND RALPH J. MOORE, JR.*

Introduction

Because your child has epilepsy, she has many rights that you need to know about. These rights, which include the right to a free appropriate public education, are provided by federal, state, and local laws. They may be essential in helping your child reach her potential by opening the door to education and special services. Epilepsy affects every child differently, and the various laws may therefore apply differently. Understanding how these laws can ensure that your child receives all the services she needs is crucial for you as the parent of a child with epilepsy.

In addition to the laws providing educational services to children who need services, there are other laws–such as those dealing with driver's licenses, discrimination, and insurance–that can affect both you and your child. These laws differ from state to state. This chapter reviews the basic principles under these types of laws.

It would be impossible to discuss the law of every state or locality. Instead, we provide an overview of the most important legal concepts

---

* Ralph J. Moore, Jr. and James E. Kaplan are attorneys in practice in Washington, D.C., and are active in the area of the legal rights for handicapped children. They are the co-authors of "Legal Rights and Hurdles: Being a Good Advocate for Your Child" in *Babies With Down Syndrome: A New Parents Guide* (Woodbine House, 1986). Mr. Moore is the author of *Handbook on Estate Planning for Families of Developmentally Disabled Persons in Maryland, the District of Columbia, and Virginia.*

you need to know. For information about the law in your area, contact the Epilepsy Foundation or your local EFA affiliate.

There are no federal laws that deal specifically with epilepsy. Rather, the rights of children with epilepsy are provided for in the laws and regulations for handicapped people generally. In other words, the same laws that protect all handicapped children can also protect your child. To effectively exercise your rights and fully protect your child, you should understand those laws.

Because epilepsy can sometimes cause serious lasting disabilities, some parents will have additional concern about the future—especially how to care for their child when they, the parents, are no longer alive. This chapter reviews some of the extremely important legal issues parents must face to protect their child's future. Finally, we summarize briefly the disability benefits generally available from federal and state governments after your child is grown.

You should understand that this chapter is designed to provide accurate and authoritative information about the legal aspects of having a child with epilepsy. There is much variation in federal and state laws as they relate to epilepsy. The authors and the publisher, however, are not acting as lawyers and are not rendering legal, accounting, or other professional advice. If you need legal or other advice, you should consult a competent professional.

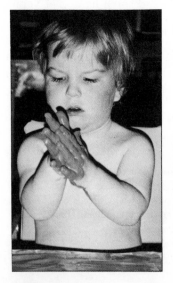

Your Child's Right To An Education

Perhaps nothing has done so much to improve the education of children with epilepsy as The Education For All Handicapped Children Act of 1975, better known as Public Law 94–142 or the EAHCA. This comprehensive law has created vastly improved educational opportunities for almost all exceptional children across the country. Administered through the Department of Education and by each state, the law works on a carrot-and-stick basis.

Under Public Law 94–142, the federal government provides funds for the education of handicapped children to each state that has a special education program that meets a variety of federal standards. To qualify for the federal funds, a state must demonstrate, through a detailed plan submitted for federal approval, that it has a policy assuring all handicapped children a "free appropriate public education." What this means is that states accepting federal funds under Public Law 94–142 must provide both approved educational services and a variety of procedural rights to handicapped children and their parents. The lure of federal funds has been attractive enough to induce all of the states to create special education plans that can truly help children with epilepsy.

The EAHCA establishes the *minimum* requirements in handicapped education programs for states wishing to receive federal funds. The federal requirements *do not require* states to adopt an ideal educational program or a program that parents feel is "the best." Because states have leeway under Public Law 94–142, there are differences from state to state in the programs or services available. Often parents perceive a difference between the federal minimum provisions and the optimum program for their child with epilepsy.

States *can* create special education programs that are better than those required by Public Law 94–142, and some have. For young children with epilepsy this is very important. Parents, organizations, and advocacy groups continually push their states to go beyond the federal requirements and provide the highest quality special education possible as early as possible. Parents should check with their local school district to find out exactly what services are available to their child.

What Public Law 94–142 Provides

The EAHCA contains many important provisions that can directly affect your child. It is worth knowing what the law says and how it works. This section reviews the important provisions of Public Law 94–142.

Coverage. Public Law 94–142 does not automatically apply to specific conditions such as epilepsy. Rather it applies to handicapped children in general. Consequently, children with epilepsy who do not need special education services are not covered. On the other hand, children who are truly handicapped by their epilepsy or the results of their seizures are entitled to special education and related services. Under the EAHCA and federal regulations, children may receive special education if it can be demonstrated that their epilepsy "adversely affects their educational performance."

Unlike other conditions, a doctor's diagnosis of epilepsy may not, by itself, be enough to establish that the EAHCA applies to your child. Parents whose children show obvious effects of epilepsy will be able to demonstrate that their child is covered. Parents whose children have impairments that are not obvious may have to convince their school district that their child needs special education services. The burden may be on you to demonstrate that this law applies to your child. How to do this effectively is discussed below. Of course, even short of EAHCA coverage, parents should work with school health and administration officials to ensure the best educational program and care for their child with epilepsy.

When Coverage Under Public Law 94–142 Begins. Generally speaking, Public Law 94–142 requires that states provide special education to handicapped children between the ages of six and eighteen. States may provide services to children between birth and age six and between ages eighteen and twenty-one, even though the EAHCA does not necessarily require it. Parents need to check with the state where they reside to determine exactly when publicly-funded services are available.

Congress recently amended Public Law 94–142 to provide for educational services at earlier ages. Beginning in 1991, states will be required to provide services to all handicapped children from the age of three. In addition, Congress has established a program of grants to support states that offer services to children from birth.

There is wide variation among the states as to when they start providing services. A few currently provide services from birth onward; some provide services at age two; most, however provide services between the ages of three and five. Unfortunately, a few states do not offer services until age six. With amendment of Public Law 94–142, however, every state will start services at age three, if not earlier.

There are many different programs available to children with handicaps in every state. In addition to Public Law 94–142, states or local school districts may provide early intervention services. There is also a federal law making grants available to local school districts for infant programs. *Even if your state does not start services under Public Law 94–142 until quite late, there may be programs available to your child now.* Check with your state department of education, your local epilepsy group, the EFA, and other parents. The Resource Guide at the end of the book contains national and state listings of agencies, organizations, and programs. Call them to find out exactly when services under Public Law 94–142 begin and what other services are available to your child now.

Length of Services. Currently under Public Law 94–142, states must provide more than the traditional 180-day school year when the unique needs of a child indicate that year-round instruction is a necessary part of a "free appropriate public education." In many states, the decision to offer summer instruction depends on whether the child will regress substantially without summer services. If so, the services must be provided at public expense.

Identification and Evaluation. Because the EAHCA applies only to handicapped children, your child must be evaluated before she is eligible for special education. Public Law 94–142 requires each state to develop testing and evaluation procedures designed to identify and evaluate the needs and abilities of each child before she is placed into a special education program. All areas of development must be tested: health, vision, hearing, social and emotional status, general intelligence, academic performance, communication ability, and motor skills. On these and other issues, the evaluation procedure is required to take into account the parents' input. That means that parents – who understand their child's developmental needs best – should take an active role in the evaluation.

As explained above, because epilepsy does not always cause handicaps, parents may have to demonstrate that their child needs special education services. If your child's epilepsy causes developmental delays or other handicaps, your school district is required to provide services. Parents should gather as much information as possible to demonstrate the need for special education. Statements or letters from doctors, evaluations by developmental specialists, and recommendations from educators can help convince your school district that your child is covered by Public Law 94–142. Never hesitate to speak up on behalf of your child's need for special education. Other parents who have been through the identification and evaluation process can be very helpful at this stage.

Learning problems, low academic achievement, and behavioral problems are some of the symptoms of epilepsy. Before a diagnosis, however, teachers and parents may not connect these symptoms with epilepsy. One of the purposes of the EAHCA is to identify children who need services as soon as possible after a problem appears. Chil-

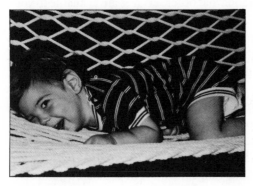

dren suffering learning and behavioral problems should be evaluated early to see if they need special education services under Public Law 94–142.

"Free Appropriate Public Education." At the heart of Public Law 94–142 is the requirement that handicapped children receive a free appropriate public education. The law defines this to mean "special education and related services." In turn, "special education" means specially designed instruction tailored to meet the unique needs of the handicapped child, including classroom instruction, physical education, home instruction, and–if necessary–instruction in hospitals or institutions. "Related services" are defined as transportation and other developmental, corrective, and supportive services necessary to enable the child to benefit from a special education. Services provided by a trained occupational therapist, physical therapist, speech therapist, psychologist, social worker, school nurse, or any other qualified person may be required under Public Law 94–142. Some services, however, are specifically excluded. Most important among these exclusions are strictly medical services that must be provided by a licensed physician or hospital.

As mentioned above, the EAHCA does not prescribe a specific educational program, but rather sets a minimum standard for the states to follow. In this way states have considerable leeway in designing special education programs. Let's examine more precisely what "free appropriate public education" means.

"Free" means that, regardless of the parents' ability to pay, every part of a child's special education program must be provided at public expense. This is true if the child is placed in a program in a public school or, if a suitable public program is not available, in a private school or residential setting. In other words, if a private school or residential placement is necessary to provide an appropriate educational program—not merely the parents' preference—then the school district must place the child in the private school and pay the tuition. In many areas, private schools have programs that are better suited to the needs of children with epilepsy. Remember, the EAHCA does not provide for tuition payment for educational services *not* approved by the school district or other governing agency (unless, as is explained elsewhere in this chapter, parents are able to overturn the decision of their school district). Parents who place their child in an unapproved program face having to bear the full cost of tuition themselves.

It often is difficult for parents to understand that the "free appropriate public education" mandated by the EAHCA does not secure for their child either the best education that money can buy or even an educational opportunity equal to that given to nonhandicapped children. The law is more modest; it only requires that handicapped children be given access to specialized educational services individually designed to benefit the handicapped child. A few years ago, the United States Supreme Court decided that a "free appropriate public education" need not be designed to enable a handicapped child to maximize his potential or to develop self-sufficiency. Instead, the basic floor of educational opportunity may be satisfied by a variety of instructional and related services, the extent of which is determined on a child-by-child basis. The law in this area is still evolving, so there are no clear rules as yet.

It is up to parents to secure the most appropriate placement and services for their child. Under the EAHCA, parents and educators are supposed to work together to design the individualized education program for each child. But to convince a school district to make the best placement for the child, parents must demonstrate to school officials not only that the school district's preferred placement might not be appropriate, but that the parents' preferred placement *is* appropriate. Hopefully in the end there is agreement on the appropriate placement. If not, there are procedures for resolving disputes that we discuss later in the chapter.

School districts are required to provide services to all handicapped children "regardless of the severity of their handicap." But if the child's handicaps are relatively minor, his special education needs are too. Consequently, the services provided will be limited. Because epilepsy is different in every child, the extent of special education services needed will be different for every child.

"Least Restrictive Environment." In discussing special education the term "mainstreaming" is often mentioned. The law requires that handicapped children must "to the maximum extent appropriate" be educated in the *least restrictive environment* with children who are *not* handicapped. Under Public Law 94–142, there is therefore a strong preference for mainstreaming handicapped children, including children with epilepsy.

In practice, the law requires that children with handicaps be integrated into their community's regular schools, if possible. For some this means a combination of special classes, along with physical education, assemblies, and other classes taken with the rest of the school. Special services and extra teaching material can be used to provide the extra educational input special children need. The law was intended to end the historical practice of isolating handicapped children.

Despite the law's preference for mainstreaming, the EAHCA also recognizes that regular classrooms may not be suitable for the education of some handicapped children. In these cases, the law allows for placement in separate classes, separate public schools, private schools, or even residential settings if this kind of placement is required to meet the individual educational—as opposed to medical, social, or emotional—needs of the child. For children for whom placement within the community's public schools is not appropriate, the law still requires that they be placed in the least restrictive educational environment suitable to their individual needs.

"Individualized Education Program." Public Law 94–142 recognizes that each handicapped child is unique. As a result, the law requires that special education programs be tailored to the individual needs of each handicapped child. Based on your child's evaluation, a program specifically designed to address her developmental problems will be devised. This is called an "individualized education program" or, more commonly, an "IEP."

The IEP is a written report that describes:

1. the child's present level of development;
2. both the short-term and annual goals of the special education program;
3. the specific educational services that the child will receive;
4. the date services will start and their expected duration;
5. standards for determining whether the goals of the educational program are being met; and
6. the extent to which the child will be able to participate in regular educational programs.

A child's IEP is usually developed during a series of meetings among the parents, teachers, and representatives of the school district. Even the child himself may be present. The effort to write an IEP is ideally a cooperative one with parents, teachers, and school officials conferring on what goals are appropriate and how best to achieve them. Preliminary drafts of the IEP are reviewed and revised until what hopefully is a mutually acceptable program is developed.

IEPs should be very detailed. Although initially this may seem intimidating, detailed IEPs enable parents to closely monitor the education their child receives and to make sure their child is actually receiving the services prescribed. In addition, the law requires that IEPs be reviewed and revised at least once a year to ensure the child's educational program continues to meet his changing needs.

Designing a suitable IEP requires direct parent involvement. You cannot always depend on teachers or school officials to recognize your child's unique needs as you do. To obtain the full range of services, you may need to demonstrate that withholding these services would result in an education that would *not* be "appropriate." For example, if parents feel a private school program is best for their child, they must demonstrate that placement in the public school program would not be appropriate for their child's special needs.

Because children with epilepsy may have special needs, it is essential that their IEP be written with care to meet those needs. Unless parents request specific services, they may be overlooked. Make sure school officials recognize the unique needs of your child–the needs that make her different from other handicapped children in general and different even from other children with epilepsy.

How can parents prepare for the IEP process? First, survey available programs, including public, private, federal, state, county, and municipal programs. Observe classes and see for yourself which program is best suited to your child. Local school districts and local organizations can provide you with information about programs in your community. Second, collect a complete set of developmental evaluations–get your own if you doubt the accuracy of the school district's evaluation. Third and most important, decide for yourself what program and services are best for your child, then request that placement.

To support placement in a particular type of program, parents can collect "evidence" that their child needs special services. Parents can support their position that a particular type of placement is appropriate by presenting letters from doctors, therapists (physical, speech, or occupational), teachers, developmental experts, and other professionals. This evidence may help persuade a school district that it would not be appropriate to deny a child the requested placement. Other suggestions to help parents through the IEP process are:

1. Don't go to placement meetings alone–bring others for support, such as spouses, doctors, teachers, and friends;
2. Keep close track of what everyone involved in your child's case is doing; and
3. *Get everything in writing.* For children with epilepsy, with their unique developmental challenges, parents need to be assertive advocates during their child's IEP process.

Resolution of Disputes under Public Law 94–142

It is usually best to resolve disputes with school districts over your child's educational program *during* the IEP process, before hard positions have been formed. Although Public Law 94–142 establishes dispute resolution procedures that are designed to be fair to parents, it is easier and far less costly to avoid disputes by coming to some agreement during the IEP process. Accordingly, our first suggestion is to try to accomplish your objectives by persuasion. If there is a dispute that simply cannot be resolved with the school district, however, this section discusses how Public Law 94–142 and other laws can be used to resolve that dispute.

In order to protect the rights of handicapped children and their parents, Public Law 94–142 establishes a variety of safeguards. For instance, prior written notice is always required for any change made in your child's identification, evaluation, or educational placement. A school district is prohibited from deceiving parents. School officials must state in writing what they want to do, when, and why.

Beyond the requirement of written notice, the EAHCA allows parents to file a formal complaint locally about *any matter* "relating to the identification, evaluation, or educational placement of the child, or the provision of free appropriate public education to such child." What this means is that parents can file a complaint about virtually any problem they may have with their child's educational program (or the refusal to provide one) if they have been unable to resolve that problem with school officials. This is a very broad right of appeal, one that parents have successfully used in the past to correct serious problems in their children's educational programs. For information about appeals, you can contact your school district, advocacy groups, and other parents. The appeal process can be started simply by filing a letter of complaint.

The first step in the appeal process is usually an "impartial due process hearing" held before a hearing examiner. This hearing, usually held on the local level, is the parents' first opportunity to explain their complaint before an impartial person who is required to listen to both sides, and then to render a decision. At the hearing, parents are entitled to be represented by an attorney or lay advocate, they can present evidence, and they can examine, cross-examine, and compel the attendance of witnesses. The child has a right to be present at the hearing as well. At the end of the hearing, parents have a right to receive a written record of the hearing, of the written findings, and of the hearing examiner's conclusions.

Just as with the IEP process, parents need to present facts that show that the school district's decisions about a child's educational program is wrong. To overturn the school district's decision, parents must show that the disputed placement does not provide their child with the "free appropriate public education" that is required by the EAHCA. Evidence in the form of letters, testimony, and expert evaluations is usually essential to a successful appeal.

Parents or school districts may appeal the decision of a hearing examiner. The appeal usually goes to the state's educational agency. This state agency is required to make an independent decision upon its review of the record of the due process hearing and of any additional evidence presented. The state agency then issues its own decision.

The right to appeal does not stop there. Parents or school officials can appeal beyond the state level by bringing a lawsuit under the EAHCA and other laws in a state or federal court. In this kind of legal action, the court must determine whether there is a preponderance of the evidence (that is, whether it is more likely than not) that the school district's placement is proper for that child. In reaching its decision, the court must give weight to the expertise of the school officials responsible for providing the child's education, but parents can and should also present their own expert evidence.

During all administrative and judicial proceedings, Public Law 94–142 requires that your child remain in her current educational placement, unless you and the local or state agencies agree to a move. Parents who unilaterally place their child in a different program risk having to bear the full cost of that program. If, however, the school district is found to have erred, it may be required to reimburse parents for the expenses of the changed placement. Accordingly, you should make a change of program only after carefully considering the potential cost of that decision.

As with any legal dispute, each phase – complaint, hearings, appeals, and court cases – can be expensive, time-consuming, and emotionally draining. As mentioned above, it is wise for you to try to resolve problems without filing a formal complaint or bringing suit. For example, you should consult with other parents who have filed complaints and should talk to sympathetic school officials. When informal means fail to resolve a problem, however, formal channels should be pursued. Your child's best interests must come first. The EAHCA grants important rights that parents need not be bashful about exercising.

Regarding expenses, parents who ultimately win their dispute with a school district may recover attorneys' fees thanks to a recent amendment to Public Law 94–142. In the past, parents had to pay their own attorneys' fees even when they won their challenge. The law was changed to allow courts, at their discretion, to award attorneys' fees to prevailing parents in cases either pending or initiated after July 3, 1984. A word of caution, however, a court can limit or refuse attorneys' fees if you reject an offer of settlement from the school district, and then do not obtain a better outcome.

The EAHCA is a powerful tool in the hands of parents. It can be used to provide unparalleled educational opportunities to children with epilepsy. Using it effectively, however, requires an understanding of how it works. The Reading List at the end of this book includes several good guidebooks to Public Law 94–142 and the special education system. With a knowledge of this vital law, parents will be far better able to help their child realize his potential.

The Rehabilitation Act Of 1973

Section 504 of the Rehabilitation Act of 1973 prohibits discrimination against qualified handicapped persons and increases their opportunities to participate in and benefit from federally-funded programs. The law provides that:

> No otherwise qualified handicapped individual . . . shall, solely by reason of his handicap, be excluded from the participation in, be denied the benefits of, or be subjected to discrimination under any program or activity receiving federal financial assistance. . . .

A handicapped individual is any person who has a physical or mental impairment that substantially limits one or more of that person's "major life activities," which consist of "caring for one's self, performing manual tasks, walking, seeing, hearing, speaking, breathing, learning, and working." The United States Supreme Court has determined that an "otherwise qualified" handicapped individual is one who is "able to meet all of a program's requirements in spite of his handicap." Programs or activities receiving federal funding must make reasonable accommodation to permit the participation of such a handicapped person.

A recent amendment to Public Law 94–142, makes it frequently possible for parents to pursue a claim against their local school district under both the EAHCA and the Rehabilitation Act. Parents must be sure, however, to first pursue all claims and appeals at the administrative level before suing under either law. As explained below, Section 504 also comes into play to assert rights beyond secondary school or rights other than those directly related to education. Prevailing parents may recover attorneys' fees under the Rehabilitation Act.

Educational Programs And Services When Your Child Is An Adult

Most children with epilepsy will be completely independent as adults. Some will have varying needs for special services depending on their particular seizure disorder and its response to treatment. Still others, because of the impact of their epilepsy, will need support and supervision in employment and daily living. This support and supervision can be provided through employment and residential programs. For example, the Epilepsy Foundation of America offers a Training and Placement Service to help people with epilepsy with vocational training and rehabilitation. In addition, in some areas there are strong movements toward noninstitutional community residential services and supported employment programs. Regrettably, if these kinds of programs are unavailable, parents are left on their own to provide the necessary support and supervision for as long as possible.

Programs vary from state to state and from community to community. As a result of state and federal budget cuts, these programs typically have long waiting lists and typically are underfunded. After your child reaches age eighteen, her right to a public education may end in many states, even though her needs may continue. Currently, the sad truth is that under Public Law 94–142 thousands of children are receiving education and training that equip them to live as independently and productively as possible, only to be sent home when they complete school with nowhere to go and nothing to do.

Now is the time to work to change this sad reality. As waiting lists grow, your child may be deprived of needed services. Because charitable funds are limited and because most families do not have the resources to pay the full cost of group homes and employment programs, the only other remedy is public funding. Just as parents banded together to demand enactment of the EAHCA, you must band together now to persuade local, state, and federal officials that our nation can afford to allow disabled people to live in dignity. Parents of handicapped *children* should not leave this job to parents of handicapped *adults*, for children become adults–all too soon.

Under the federal Developmentally Disabled Assistance and Bill of Rights Act, states which meet the law's requirements can receive grants for a variety of programs. Important among them is a protection and advocacy (P&A) system. A P&A system works to protect and advocate for the civil and legal rights of persons with developmental disabilities. People with epilepsy were originally covered expressly by this law, but a recent amendment has made eligibility for people with epilepsy more difficult. The law now requires that it be demonstrated that a person's epilepsy interferes with or prevents a person from carrying out daily activities. Because persons who are severely disabled by epilepsy cannot always protect their own rights or speak out for themselves, it is important that each state's P&A system include fair evaluation criteria for persons with epilepsy.

Vocational Training Programs

There is one educational program supported by federal funding that is available to adults with epilepsy who need it. Operating much like Public Law 94–142, there are federal laws making funds available to support vocational training and rehabilitation. Again, states wanting federal funds must submit plans for approval. Federal law provides that all people who have a mental disability that constitutes a "substantial handicap to employment" and who can be expected to benefit from vocational services are eligible. Unlike the EAHCA, however, handicapped individuals are not granted enforceable rights and procedures under these laws.

The state Departments of Vocational Rehabilitation are sometimes called "DVR" or "Voc Rehab." People who apply for Voc Rehab services are evaluated and an "Individualized Written Rehabilitation Plan," similar to an IEP, is developed. Under these programs, adults with epilepsy can continue to receive vocational education after they reach age twenty-one. Parents should contact their state vocational rehabilitation department or the EFA for specific information on services available to their child with epilepsy. Despite shrinking federal and state budgets, some states and communities offer their own programs, such as group homes, supported employment programs, and life-skills classes. Contact other parents and organizations.

Driver's Licenses

As your child with epilepsy approaches the age at which she will want to start driving, you will need to understand the laws of your state regulating driving by people with epilepsy. Currently, all states have

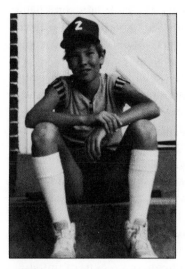

regulations of one kind or another, but these regulations are so varied that it is important for you to check with your department of motor vehicles. They should be able to provide you with a booklet explaining your state's laws.

The most common of the driver's license regulations is that a person with epilepsy be free of seizures for between six and twelve months before obtaining a license. The trend in the law is toward a shorter seizure-free period. Most states require the submission of medical reports to the state department of motor vehicles from time to time so they can monitor a driver's current condition.

Some states do not require a seizure-free period at all. Instead, they rely on doctor's statements about a person's ability to drive safely. This is preferable to seizure free periods because it treats people with epilepsy individually based on their ability to drive. Other states place restrictions on licenses that limit driving to the daytime, driving to and from work, driving in emergencies, or during certain hours. Many states have appeal procedures for people who have been rejected for a driver's license or have had restrictions placed on it. Check with your local department of motor vehicles, your neurologist, local organizations, and the EFA's toll free number about the regulations in your state.

Employment And Other Discrimination

When your child is older, employment becomes quite important. Too often, people with epilepsy are denied employment out of a fear of their potential seizures, even when those seizures are controlled medically. Because people with epilepsy can suffer discrimination as a result of their condition, it is important for you to understand the laws that deal with this problem. There are a wide variety of both state and federal laws that deal with discrimination against people with handicaps. This section provides an overview of those laws; contact your state anti-discrimination agency or the EFA for information about your state's laws.

Just about every state has its own law prohibiting employment discrimination on the basis of handicap, although these laws vary tremendously and can be quite ineffective. If someone is capable of performing a job, the law makes it illegal to deny employment because that person has a handicap. Some states specifically mention epilepsy or neurological conditions in their definition of a handicap.

It is usually up to persons claiming discrimination to demonstrate that their condition is not a barrier to employment; that they could perform the duties of their job adequately despite their epilepsy. Because employment discrimination is often the result of fear of seizures – rather than actual seizures – most people with epilepsy know they can perform most jobs as well as other people. The law prohibits employers from using the mere existence of the condition to deny employment.

When is it permissible to deny employment on the basis of epilepsy and when is it not? Because every job has different duties and every person with epilepsy has different symptoms (some effectively have none), there are no clear-cut rules. If a person's epilepsy does not cause substantial interference with job performance, it is usually unlawful to deny employment on that basis. Sometimes freedom from a condition is stated as a qualification for a job, but these restrictions should be based on reality, not outdated notions and stereotypes. In addition, some states prohibit pre-employment inquiries which are unrelated to an applicant's suitability. In these states, an employer is not allowed to ask a person about epilepsy and an applicant does not have to mention his epilepsy unless it affects job performance or safety. Some states provide for medical examinations to determine the impact of a person's epilepsy on job performance. Finally, some states have requirements that employers attempt to make "reasonable accommodations"—a term left vague by the courts—for the handicapped so that employers cannot deny employment because someone's epilepsy causes trivial employment consequences.

There are state agencies charged with enforcing the anti-discrimination laws. If you or your child feel that she has been discriminated against, most states provide for filing a complaint with the state agency first. These agencies can investigate complaints, attempt to negotiate a settlement, hold hearings, and issue decisions. You have the right to appeal to the courts if you are dissatisfied with an agency's decision. Be sure to contact your state anti-discrimination agency or the EFA for assistance in pursuing a claim of discrimination.

In addition to state laws, the Rehabilitation Act of 1973 prohibits discrimination on the basis of handicaps in the federal government, by federal contractors, and in federally-funded programs. Many of the state laws are patterned after on the Rehabilitation Act—they have similar provisions such as the "reasonable accommodation" requirement and the prohibition of pre-employment inquiries. A variety of federal agencies are responsible for enforcing this law: 1) complaints against a federal government agency must be filed with the Equal Employment Opportunity Commission; 2)complaints against a contractor doing business with the federal government must be filed with Office of Federal Contract Compliance Programs of the Department of Labor; and 3) complaints against an organization receiving federal funds must be filed with the civil rights office of the federal agency providing the funds. Complaints of discrimination must be filed with the appropriate federal agency before any lawsuit can be brought. You should understand that, in some cases, both state law *and* the Rehabilitation Act can be used to combat employment discrimination. There are organizations and attorneys specializing in this area of law.

Children with epilepsy can also suffer from discrimination. Sometimes the fear of epilepsy—rather than any actual disability—results in restrictions. Physical activities at school or eligibility for camping can sometimes be denied on the basis of epilepsy alone. The Rehabilitation Act and some state laws can be used to challenge this discrimination. Children should not be denied activities if their epilepsy does not pose a danger; these laws can help. Check with the EFA for information about the laws in your state.

Insurance

For many families with a child with epilepsy, insurance can be a serious problem. The fact is that most insurance companies will not offer health, life, and automobile coverage at reasonable rates to persons with epilepsy. This is a result of the belief that children and adults with epilepsy are likely to have more claims submitted than others. These practices have persisted despite the gains in the treatment of epilepsy that allow many people to achieve seizure control.

About half the states have laws that outlaw handicap-based discrimination by prohibiting insurance companies from using a handicap such as epilepsy as an excuse to decline coverage. The drawback to these laws, however, is that they allow insurance companies to decline coverage if the denial is based on "sound actuarial principles" or "actual or reasonable anticipated loss experience." Insurers rely on these provisions to deny coverage, claiming that people with epilepsy submit more claims. The laws, in short, are not very effective in protecting families from insurance discrimination.

Some states have attempted to ease the automobile insurance burden for families by offering assigned risk insurance plans. These plans assign "higher risk" drivers to insurance companies so that everyone has automobile insurance coverage. Although the insurance rates are higher, these plans at least offer coverage. Check with your department of motor vehicles, state insurance commission, or the EFA for information about assigned risk automobile insurance in your area.

In the area of health insurance, a few states have begun to offer shared risk health insurance plans. These plans work like assigned risk automobile insurance: they offer coverage to people who could not get coverage otherwise. The added cost is shared among all insurance companies (including HMOs) operating in the state. To be eligible, a person must show that he has been recently turned down for coverage or offered a policy with limited coverage. Some laws also cover people who have received premium increases of fifty percent. As with assigned risk automobile insurance, the cost of this kind of health insurance is usually higher, but it usually is better than no health insurance at all. Again, check with your state insurance commission and the EFA for information about health insurance programs in your area.

Planning for Your Child's Future

Although the overwhelming majority of children with epilepsy grow into independent adults, there is a significant minority for whom epilepsy is a lifelong serious disability. This section of the book is for the parents of those children.

The possibility that your child may be dependent all of her life can be overwhelming. To meet your child's future needs, you need information in areas you may never have thought about before and you must find inner resources you may not believe exist. In most families, parents remain primarily responsible for ensuring their child's well-being. Consequently, questions that deeply trouble parents include: "What will happen to my child when I die? Who will look after her? How will her financial needs be met?"

Some parents of children with epilepsy delay dealing with these issues, coping instead with the immediate demands of the present. Others begin to address the future. They add to their insurance, begin (alone or with grandparents) to set aside funds for their child, and share with family and friends their concerns about their child's future needs. Whatever the course, parents need to understand in advance some serious problems that affect planning for a disabled child's future. Failure to avoid these pitfalls can have dire future consequences for your child and for other family members.

There are three important issues that families of children with disabling epilepsy need to consider in planning for the future. These are:

1. the potential for cost-of-care liability;
2. the complex rules governing eligibility for government benefits; and

3. the child's ability to handle her own affairs.

Of course, there are many other matters that may be different for parents of special children. For example, insurance needs may be affected, and the important choice of trustees and guardians is more difficult. But these types of concerns face most parents in one form or another. Cost-of-care liability, government benefits, and the inability to manage one's own affairs, however, present issues that are unique to the parents of handicapped children.

Cost-of-Care Liability

When a state provides residential services to a handicapped person, it usually has the power to force that person to pay for them. Called "cost-of-care liability," this power allows states to tap the handicapped person's own funds to pay for the services the state provides.

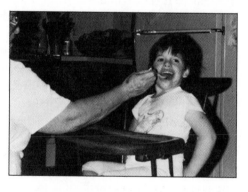

States can reach funds owned outright by a handicapped person and even funds set aside in some trusts. A few states go further. Some impose liability on parents for the care of an adult handicapped person; and some impose liability for other services in addition to residential care. This is an area parents need to look into early and carefully.

The most unfortunate and seemingly unfair aspect of cost-of-care liability is that these payments do *not* benefit the handicapped person. Ordinarily they add nothing to the care and services the individual receives. Instead, the money is deposited into the general funds of the state to pay for roads, schools, public officials' salaries, and so on.

It is natural for parents to want to pass their worth on to their child through their wills or through gifts. The unfortunate effect of allowing a child with epilepsy to inherit a portion of your estate, however, may be the same as naming the state in your will—something most people would not do voluntarily. Similarly, setting aside funds in your child's name, in a support trust, or in a Uniform Gifts to Minors Act (UGMA) account may be the same as giving money to the state, money that could better be used to meet the future needs of your child.

What, then, can parents do? The specific answer depends on circumstances and the law of your state. Here are three basic strategies parents use:

First, strange as it may seem, in some cases the best solution is to disinherit a child with disabling epilepsy, leaving funds instead to siblings in the clear hope that they will use these funds for their disabled sibling's benefit, even though they will be under *no* legal obligation to do so. The absence of a legal obligation is crucial. It protects the funds from cost-of-care claims. The state will simply have no basis for claiming that the handicapped person owns the funds. This strategy, however, runs the risk that the funds will not be used for your child with epilepsy if the siblings: 1)choose not to use them that way; 2)suffer financial reversals or domestic problems of their own, exposing the funds to creditors or spouses; or 3) die without making arrangements that safeguard the funds.

A second method used in states where the law is favorable to this arrangement is to leave funds intended for the benefit of your child with disabling epilepsy in what is called a "discretionary" trust. This kind of trust is created to supplement, rather than replace, state benefits. Under discretionary trusts, the trustee (the person in charge of the trust assets) has the power to use or not use the trust funds for any purpose, although the funds can only be used for the benefit of the handicapped child. In many states, these types of trusts are not subject to cost-of-care claims because the trust does not impose any legal obligation on the trustee to spend funds for care and support. In contrast, "support" trusts *require* the trustee to use the funds for the care and support of the child and can be subjected to state cost-of-care claims. Discretionary trusts can be created under your will or during your lifetime, but, as with all legal documents, must be carefully written. In some states, to protect the trust against cost-of-care claims, it is necessary to add provisions to such a trust stating clearly that it is to be used to supplement rather than supplant publicly funded services and benefits.

A third method to avoid cost-of-care claims is to create a trust, either under your will or during your lifetime, that describes the kind of allowable expenditures to be made for your handicapped child in a way that excludes care in state-funded programs. Like discretionary trusts, these trusts – sometimes called "luxury" trusts – are intended to supplement, rather than take the place of, state benefits. The state cannot reach these funds because the trust forbids spending any funds on care in state institutions.

In using all of these estate planning techniques, parents should consult a qualified attorney who is experienced in estate planning for parents of handicapped children. Because each state's laws differ and because each family has unique circumstances, individualized estate planning is essential.

Eligibility for Government Benefits

There are a wide variety of federal, state, and local programs for handicapped persons. Each of these programs provides different services and each has its own complex eligibility requirements. What parents and grandparents do now to provide financially for their child with epilepsy can have important effects on that child's eligibility for government assistance in the future.

There are four major federally-funded programs that can help people with disabling epilepsy. First, "Supplemental Security Income" (SSI), a public assistance program, and "Social Security Disability Insurance" (SSDI), a disability insurance program, can both be applicable to people with epilepsy that incapacitates them for work. Both are designed to provide a monthly income to qualified disabled persons.

Under current rules, it can be difficult for people with epilepsy to qualify as "disabled." It must be shown that a person's epilepsy is so disabling that he cannot be gainfully employed and that it amounts to a "severe" medical impairment. This impairment must limit the person's ability to perform basic work activities, such as walking, standing, and lifting.

The eligibility requirements, however, do not end there. SSDI is not based on financial need. Instead, eligibility is based on the disabled's own work record prior to disability or on a retired or deceased parent's social security coverage in the case of persons disabled before age eighteen. On the other hand, eligibility for SSI is based on financial need, and thus an applicant's resources and other income can disqualify him from receiving SSI. Remember, what your child owns in her own name and what income she is entitled to receive under a trust can prevent her from receiving these government benefits.

Medicare and Medicaid are also potentially important to people with epilepsy, but each has its own eligibility requirements. Medicaid provides medical assistance to persons who are eligible for SSI and to other people with incomes deemed insufficient to pay for medical care. Because eligibility is based on financial need, placing assets in the name of a child with epilepsy or providing that child with income through a trust can disqualify the child. Medicare, however, is not based on financial need. Instead, persons entitled to receive benefits under Social Security are entitled to Medicare payments.

It is important for parents to become generally familiar with the rules governing SSI, SSDI, Medicaid, and Medicare. It is even more important to avoid an unwitting mistake that could disqualify your child from receiving these benefits. If your child may be disabled as an adult, do not set aside funds in your child's own name, create a support trust, or establish a custodial account under the Uniform Gifts to Minors Act UGMA (discussed below). Follow the type of strategies outlined above. You will need competent professional assistance, of course, because these are quite technical matters.

Competence to Manage Financial Affairs

Even if your child with epilepsy may never need state-funded residential care or government benefits, it is possible she will need help in handling her financial affairs throughout her life. In this event, care must be exercised in giving assets to your child. To do this, there are a wide variety of trusts that can allow someone else to control the ways in which money is spent after you die. Of course, the amount of financial control depends on many different circumstances, such as your child's capacity to manage assets properly, her relationship with her siblings, and your financial status. Each family's situation is different. A knowledgeable attorney can review the various alternatives and help you to pick the one best suited to your family.

Estate Planning for Parents of Children With Disabling Epilepsy

More than most parents, the parents of a child with severe epilepsy need to attend to estate planning. Because of cost-of-care liability, government benefits, and competency concerns, it is vital that you make plans. Parents need to name the people who will care for their special child in the event of the parents' deaths. They need to review their insurance to be sure it is adequate in light of their child's special needs. They need to make sure their retirement plans are arranged to help their disabled child's education and training beyond the age of eighteen. They need to inform grandparents of cost-of-care liability, government benefits, and competency problems to make sure the grandparents do not inadvertently waste resources that could otherwise benefit their grandchild's future. Most of all, they need to make a will so that their hopes and plans are realized and so that the disastrous consequences of dying without a will are avoided.

Proper estate planning differs for each family. Every will needs to be tailored to individual needs. There are no formula wills, especially for parents of a child with severe epilepsy. There are, however, some common mistakes to avoid. Here is a list:

No Will. If parents die without first making wills, the law generally requires that each child in the family share equally in the parents' estate. The result is that your child with disabling epilepsy will inherit property in her own name. If her epilepsy is severe, her inheritance may become subject to cost-of-care claims and could jeopardize eligibility for government benefits. These and other problems can be avoided with a properly drafted will. Parents should never allow the state to determine how their property will be divided upon their death. Planning can make you feel uneasy, but it is too important to ignore.

A Will Leaving Property Outright to the Child With Disabling Epilepsy. Like having no will at all, a will that leaves property to a handicapped child in his own name may subject the inheritance to cost-of-care liability and may risk disqualifying him from government benefits. Parents of children with severe epilepsy do not just need any will, they need a will that meets their special needs.

A Will Creating a Support Trust for the Child With Disabling Epilepsy. A will that creates a support trust presents much the same problem as a will that leaves property outright to the child with severe epilepsy. The funds in these trusts may be subject to cost-of-care claims and jeopardize government benefits. Have a will drafted that avoids this problem.

Insurance and Retirement Plans Naming the Child With Disabling Epilepsy as a Beneficiary. Many parents own life insurance policies or maintain retirement plans that name a handicapped child as a beneficiary or contingent beneficiary, either alone or in common with siblings. The result: funds may go outright to your child with disabling epilepsy, creating cost-of-care liability and government benefits eligibility problems. Parents of such a child should designate the funds to go to someone else or to go into a properly drawn trust.

Use of Joint Tenancy in Lieu of Wills. Spouses sometimes avoid making wills by placing all their property in joint tenancies. In joint tenancies, property is owned equally by each spouse; when one spouse dies, the survivor automatically becomes the sole owner. Parents try to use joint tenancies instead of wills, relying on the surviving spouse to properly take care of all estate planning matters. This plan, however, fails completely if both parents die in a common disaster, if the surviving spouse becomes incapacitated, or if the surviving spouse neglects to make a proper will. The result is the same as if neither spouse made any will at all—the child with epilepsy shares equally in the parents' estates. If the condition is disabling, this may expose the assets to cost-of-care liability and give rise to problems with government benefits. Therefore, even when all property is held by spouses in joint tenancy, it is necessary that both spouses make wills.

Establishing UGMA Accounts for the Child With Potentially Disabling Epilepsy. Over and over again well-meaning parents and grandparents of handicapped children set up accounts under the Uniform Gift to Minors Act (UGMA). When the child reaches age eighteen or twenty-one, the account becomes the property of the child. Once again, problems may arise with cost-of-care liability and with eligibility for Medicaid or SSI, just at the time those benefits may be needed to help pay for adult services and programs. Parents should *never* establish UGMA accounts for their child with severe epilepsy nor should they open other bank accounts in the child's name.

Failing to Advise Grandparents and Relatives of the Need for Special Arrangements. Just as the parents of a handicapped child properly drafted wills or trusts, so do grandparents and other relatives who may leave (or give) property to the child. If these persons are not aware of the special concerns – cost-of-care liability, government benefits, and competency – their generosity may go awry and may foil the best laid plans of the child's parents. Make sure anyone planning gifts or bequests to your child with disabling epilepsy understands what is at stake.

Children and adults with epilepsy are entitled to lead full and rewarding lives. To do so, they need proper financial support. Planning for the future *now* is the best way to assure they will have that support when they need it. Doing otherwise can tragically shortchange their future.

Conclusion

Parenthood brings responsibilities many people never considered beforehand. Extra responsibilities confront parents of a child with epilepsy. You need to know and assert your child's rights to guarantee that she will receive the education and government benefits to which she is entitled. Similarly, understanding the pitfalls of not planning for the future and taking steps to avoid these pitfalls help parents to meet their special responsibilities. Being a good advocate for your child requires more than knowledge; you must also be determined to use that knowledge effectively and, when necessary, forcefully.

REFERENCES

Burgdorf, R. & Spicer, P. *The Legal Rights of Handicapped Persons.* Baltimore: Paul H. Brookes Publishing Co. 1980 & Supp. 1983.

Herr, S., Arons, S. & Wallace, R. Jr. *Legal Rights and Mental-Health Care.* Lexington, MA: D.C. Heath & Co. 1983.

Herr, S. *Rights and Advocacy for Retarded People.* Lexington, MA: D.C. Heath & Company 1983.

Rothstein, L. *Rights of Physically Handicapped Persons.* New York: McGraw-Hill Book Co. 1984 & Supp. 1986.

Children With Special Needs. Law and Contemporary Problems. Vol. 48, Parts 1 & 2, Winter and Spring 1985.

Parent Statements

Parents get to the placement meeting and are told by the school officials, "Your child's needs aren't severe enough to require a private placement." They use that tone so the parents think, "Oh great, he doesn't need that class we thought he needed." So they stick 'em in a class with too many kids. And the parents walk out feeling relieved. It saves the school district a lot of money. Where's the advocate to help these parents realize that it's their legal right to ask for other things?

We've given a lot to charitable causes, probably more than most people. But they've not helped us. The education he receives is because of the law – not because of open hearts.

One of the things that we have been through lately was setting up a trust fund and wills and things like that. The biggest problem is how do you provide for Matthew forever without making the others feel like you have stripped away providing for them. That's only in a monetary sense but it really carries over to all aspects of our time. We concentrate far more on being fair than we ever would if everything were normal.

How can the siblings be best set up to take their best shot at life, without depriving Matthew of lifetime care? We were told that he'd live a normal life span – so figure thirty or so years after me. So the proper balancing of resources and time is a major, major factor. More than we'd ever tinker with if our children were all normal.

We're making a will to provide for her in case she's not able to provide for herself. We also have to find those special people to take care of our children should anything happen to my husband and me. People who can deal with Kirsten's epilepsy. Not an easy task.

We realized soon after Ray's school began that we had to provide private therapy. The public program just couldn't meet our definition of appropriate. Speech therapy was provided in ten minute spurts throughout the week. He really needed to have the sixty minutes in one hour sessions.

Everything we learned about PL 94–142 was after the fact. After mistakes were made. I wish we had a parent support group to deal with special education and related services. It would have saved us so much time and wasted energy.

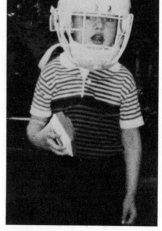

Sometimes I think about his future. When I am sixty-five, he'll just be twenty-eight. He'll live long after me and I want him to be taken care of. We're planning for his future even though we dread the thought of it.

We haven't planned one bit for our son's future. We're just taking one day at a time.

It is endlessly upsetting to face a special education placement each year. It means advocating for your kid's rights over and over again.

Our first IEP was general and had no measurable goals. Our son drifted through that first year meeting goals like "improve daily living skills." Unfortunately we had an inappropriate placement and we had to appeal. We even called the state's Department of Education to let them know we weren't receiving services. It turned out they needed to hear from people like us so they could substantiate more funding for programs.

My advice to other parents is to find an attorney and become friends. Bring him or her into your team and try to work together for the greater benefit of your family's future.

When you have a normal kid you think of college funds and then your thinking kind of stops for them and you say, "Now let us grow old together." With our situation, our thinking has to go on forever and then past us.

NINE

— ❊ —

Legislative Advocacy

THE HONORABLE TONY COELHO
UNITED STATES HOUSE OF REPRESENTATIVES*

When I was fifteen, I received a head injury and a year later began having seizures. Different doctors thought my seizures were caused by different things and I was treated in all kinds of ways but they never figured out what it was. I wasn't properly diagnosed until I was preparing to graduate from college.

People's reactions hurt me; even my parents denied the reality of epilepsy. They said no son of theirs was an epileptic, that I had to get away from those crazy friends of mine and come home. Only years later did I learn that there was a Portuguese superstition – and I'm 100 percent Portuguese – that epilepsy means possession by the Devil.

For years I hesitated to tell people I had epilepsy but when I entered public life I decided to bring it out in the open. I had been learning as much as I could about epilepsy and felt that it was time to do what I could to help dispel the myths about it. I have tried in many ways to become a public figure who works on behalf of all of us who have epilepsy. That is why I have written this chapter so that you can work with me toward a brighter future for all of us.

---

* Tony Coelho is the former House Majority whip in the United States House of Representatives.

Advocacy Means Getting Involved

Advocacy is a valuable tool in educating the public about epilepsy. As you know, many citizens, including public officials, either don't know anything about epilepsy, or are misinformed. Many parents that I have talked to don't understand how they can be effective advocates. They believe that advocacy is only for lawyers or experts. Nothing

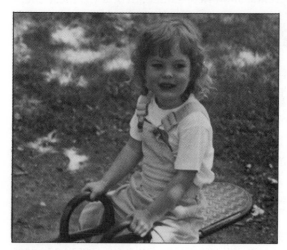

could be further from the truth! You are the expert on your child and are often in the best position to communicate his or her needs.

Parents can engage in many types of advocacy. Every time you speak out to secure services or to protect your child's rights, you are acting as an advocate. In addition to being an advocate for your child, you can also have a major impact by advocating for legislative or regulatory change at the state and national level. This type of advocacy can help not only your child, but hundreds of thousands of children with epilepsy and other disabilities.

This chapter will give you some helpful hints to become an effective legislative advocate. The methods I discuss for working with the U.S. Congress can also be useful in educating state, county, and municipal legislators. Each legislative body will have its own variations in protocol. Thus, it's important to become familiar with differences in your own state government.

As you have seen from the previous chapter, many federal and state laws affect your child—in education, access to health care, insurance, and civil rights. Public Law 94–142 (The Education for All Handicapped Children Act) and Section 504 of the Rehabilitation Act of 1973 are the primary laws affecting children with disabilities.

Public Law 94–142 exists in part because thousands of parents of children with epilepsy and other disabilities realized that their children deserved the right to be educated in the public school system and fought for that right. Similarly, the well-stated concerns of parents and individuals with disabilities were part of the impetus for the passage of Section 504 and its subsequent amendments.

I believe that parental and/or consumer advocacy is most effective when it is well focused on a particular issue. However, I don't believe that parents should work solely on issues that only affect children with disabilities. You need to think ahead to the services your child may need down the road. For example, laws which protect against employment discrimination while not essential for a child, are critical for adults. Thus, it is just as important for you to advocate on behalf of laws prohibiting employment discrimination as it is to advocate for special education.

The following few pages will give you an overview of the legislative process and the role of advocates. Once you understand the process you can see how easy it is to be an effective advocate.

The Legislative Process

How a Bill Becomes Law

To advocate effectively it is necessary to understand how the legislative process works. These are the basic steps of how a bill moves through Congress:

1. A bill is drafted.
2. A member of Congress introduces the bill with other members as original co-sponsors, the bill is then assigned a number, and referred to the appropriate committee. The member and original co-sponsors encourage their colleagues to co-sponsor the bill.
3. The committee refers the bill to one of its subcommittees.
4. The subcommittee will then hold hearings on the bill.
5. The subcommittee conducts reviews of the bill in a "markup" session, at which it makes changes if necessary and

considers amendments. If the committee adopts the bill, it sends it to the full committee for consideration.

6. The full committee holds hearings, conducts a mark-up, makes changes if necessary, adopts it, and sends or "reports" it to the full House or Senate for consideration. (House bills must first be cleared by the Rules Committee, where debate times are often established.)

7. The House and Senate debate the bill. Additional amendments are considered at this time, and the bill is either adopted or defeated.

8. If both sides adopt the bill, members of the House and Senate meet in a "Conference" to reconcile differences in their respective versions of the bill and write a Conference Report.

9. The Conference Report, containing the compromise version of the bill, is submitted to both the House and Senate and adopted.

10. The bill is sent to the White House for presidential action. If the President signs it, it becomes law. If he vetoes it, both the House and Senate, by roll-call votes of two-thirds, must agree to override the veto.

This process is followed for all legislation. It is important to understand that there are three major types of legislation—new bills, reauthorization bills, and appropriations bills.

New bills create programs or rights. Bills are developed because of impetus from many different sources. For example, some bills may be introduced in response to court decisions. The Handicapped Children Protection Act, which authorizes parents to be reimbursed for their attorneys' fees and court costs in judicial and administrative hearings under P.L. 94–142, was introduced in response to a Supreme Court decision which held that such payments were not allowed under the then existing laws. (From my perspective, the reason this bill passed was that thousands of parents let their legislators know how important its passage was to them and their children.)

Most legislation creating programs for children with disabilities, such as The Education for All Handicapped Children Act and the Rehabilitation Act, must be reauthorized every few years or the programs will end. When Congress considers a bill to reauthorize a program, it evaluates how effective the program has been, through hearings and information received from parents, consumers, other advocates, service providers, and other professionals.

Congress can either curtail or expand programs in reauthorization bills. For example, in the 1986 bill which reauthorized The Education for All Handicapped Children Act (P.L. 94–142), Congress significantly expanded the Act by creating a major new program for early intervention services for infants with disabilities from birth through age two.

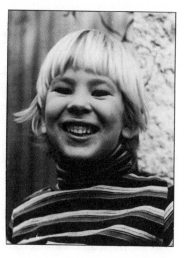

A bill authorizing a program establishes a maximum level of funding for each fiscal year. However, the program will not take effect unless and until an appropriations bill passes earmarking funds for it. For example, in 1986, Congress passed the Temporary Child Care for Handicapped Children and Crisis Nurseries Act as part of the Children's Justice Act. This Act was intended to establish demonstration programs for respite care services. Respite care is designed to alleviate the stress experienced by parents caring for disabled children on a twenty-four hour basis, by providing temporary nonmedical child care for those children. Since no money was appropriated in 1986 for this program, the program has not yet taken effect.

The federal appropriations bill of most importance to epilepsy is the one covering the Departments of Labor, Health and Human Services, and Education. This bill sets funding levels for the National Institute of Neurological and Communicative Disorders and Stroke (NINCDS), the arm of the National Institutes of Health which conducts epilepsy research. In addition, programs for respite care, special education, vocational rehabilitation, and job training receive funds from this bill.

As you can see, appropriations bills are as important as the bills originally authorizing programs, especially in these times of deficit reduction. It is crucial for parents and other advocates to voice their concerns to members of the Appropriations Committees of both Houses. If your Senator or Representative does not sit on this committee, you can still write him or her a letter and ask that your concerns be conveyed to the chairman of the Appropriations Committee.

You can obtain a copy of a bill or a committee report by writing to:

House Document Room
H-226 Capitol
Washington, D.C. 20515
Phone 202/225–3456

Senate Document Room
SH B 04
Washington, D.C. 20510
Phone 202/224–7860

Always identify the bill or report by number. Your Member's office can also assist you in getting these documents.

To find out the status of a bill, you can call the Congressional Status Office at 202/225–1772. You must provide either the number or title of the bill that you are interested in.

You may be wondering how you can find out which bills are important for people with disabilities. In addition to media sources such as newspapers and television, many disability organizations publicize information about important legislation in their newsletters. The Epilepsy Foundation of America's *National Spokesman* contains monthly reports on pending legislation in Congress. In addition, the foundation's affiliates can provide you with information about important state and local legislation.

The Role of Advocates in this Process

Advocates play an important role at all stages of the legislative process. Ideas for legislation evolve from many sources. Frequently, a member will introduce a bill after hearing of his/her constituents' needs or problems. For example, the Temporary Child Care for Handicapped Children and Crisis Nurseries Act was introduced after parents of children with severe disabilities contacted Representative George Miller of California, Chairman of the Select Committee on Children, Youth and Families, and told him of the urgent need for these services. In addition, parent groups were consulted as the legislation was drafted. This program will ultimately be funded if many other Members hear from parents in their districts about the need for respite care.

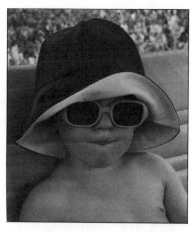

The Family and Medical Leave Act, which is now pending in Congress, is another example of the importance of parental input at all stages of the legislative process. This bill, which gives parents unpaid leave from their jobs for the birth, adoption, or serious health condition of their children, evolved out of a desire of parents to be with the newborn or newly adopted child without risking the loss of their job and a recognition by policy makers of the growing numbers of working mothers in this country.

Groups representing parents of children with disabilities and chronic health conditions came forward and urged the bill's chief sponsors to provide parental leave for a child's serious health condition as well. I became an original co-sponsor of this legislation specifically because the bill addresses the needs of parents of children with epilepsy and other disabilities. Other members have also become co-sponsors after hearing of the dilemmas faced by parents in their districts who have to work to support their families, but need time off when their children are hospitalized or undergoing medical treatment.

Parents have testified on the need for this legislation at hearings in Washington and across the country at regional field hearings. One parent of a three year old with epilepsy told a House Committee how she was given an ultimatum by her employer while her son was hospitalized in serious condition, to either show up for work or quit her job. Her testimony and that of several other parents has been the most powerful demonstration of the need of this legislation.

Testifying at hearings is not only an excellent way to educate Members of Congress about epilepsy but it also provides an opportunity to educate the public. Frequently the press will report on testimony given during hearings. For example, after the mother referred to above testified on the Family and Medical Leave Act, there were many newspaper stories published across the country that told her story.

Other parents who have similar stories but are unable to come to Washington to testify can write their statements and have them submitted for the hearing record. Members of Congress always want to hear from people who would be affected by pending legislation to emphasize the urgent need to pass the legislation.

Parents also have an opportunity to be heard when a bill is being debated on the floor before a vote. If Members have received strong letters of support or have heard stories from their constituents, they will frequently read those statements on the floor. In my opinion, floor statements that discuss the human element of a bill are the most persuasive. These statements are reprinted in the Congressional Record and become part of the law's legislative history.

Parent groups will work with Committee staffs to educate committee members, and they will be consulted if compromise language is drafted. Before the bill goes to the floor, it will be crucial for Members to receive as many letters and calls as possible urging them to vote for the bill. The communication a Member receives from his/her district on this bill will, in many cases, determine how he/she will vote.

Coalitions: The Key to Effective Advocacy

Working with other parents in coalitions is the real key to effective advocacy. There is strength in numbers! You should work within your own parent support group – develop a list of each family's legislators, at the state and national level for targeting purposes. Discuss pending legislation at meetings. Work with other parent groups and epilepsy affiliates in your state. Working in coalitions with other disability groups is absolutely critical. You will find that you share many concerns with parents of children with other disabilities.

Some initiatives require forming or working with a broader coalition. For example, over two hundred national organizations, representing people with epilepsy and other disabilities, women, the elderly, and minorities have joined in a united coalition to pass the Civil Rights Restoration Act of 1987. This bill will ensure that institutions receiving federal funds will not be able to use tax dollars to discriminate on the basis of race, sex, age, or handicap. This is critical civil rights legislation for people with epilepsy. Its ultimate success will be due to the strength and cohesiveness of this coalition.

Epilepsy advocates across the country are now beginning to work with other health, disability, children's, and low income groups on issues like access to affordable health care. In the past, coalitions of epilepsy and other disability groups, consumer safety advocates, and the insurance industry have worked together successfully to enact mandatory seat belt laws in many states.

The Nuts And Bolts Of Advocacy

Meetings with Legislators

All members of Congress have offices in their districts as well as in Washington. You don't have to travel to Washington to be effective! To arrange a meeting with a Representative or Senator, call the Member's office and ask to speak with the administrative aide in charge of appointments. Explain who you are and why you and/or your group want to meet with the Member. The administrative aide may set up a meeting for you with the Member's legislative aide who handles the issue of concern to you.

If you are not close to Washington, meet with your Representative, Senator, or their staffs in their district offices. Information from district staff on meetings with constituents is always conveyed to the Member in Washington. Some Members hold open office hours during Congressional recesses. Others hold Town Page Meetings or Citizens' Forums in their districts. Use these gatherings to get to know your Member and educate him on what pending legislation will affect children with epilepsy.

Don't wait until you have a problem to meet with your legislator. It's important to educate them about your issues. A good way to enhance their understanding about epilepsy and your child's needs is to invite him/her to visit programs that provide needed services for your child when he/she is back home. For example, ask them to tour a demonstration/pilot program which could be implemented if funding were available. Seeing an early intervention or job training program first hand is invaluable for Members. Show them your success stories as well as programs with shortcomings. Also invite them to speak to your parent group. Don't feel offended if the Member can't attend and offers to send a staff member.

Always take advantage of your opportunities to educate a Congressional staff person. Legislative aides are a Member's right hand on issues – they prepare all the documentation and briefing material, and advise Members on whether or not to support a bill. Like other members of Congress, I depend on my staff to provide me with background information on issues.

When you meet with a Member or his/her staff, always be well prepared. Focus on one issue if possible. Always describe *exactly* what you want him/her to do – vote for or against a bill, introduce a bill, make a speech, talk to another Member. Know your subject. Tell the Member or staff person exactly how the legislation will affect your child and others in his/her district. Bring along any documentation you have to help you make your case – fact sheets, surveys, reports, newspaper articles, or photographs.

Offer to assemble any other information the Member may need. Always follow up a meeting with a Member or staff person with a letter summarizing your discussion and your position on an issue. And always write a thank-you letter to the Member or legislative aide.

Letters

The easiest and most effective way to communicate with a Member or Congress or other elected official is by letter. I receive an average of six hundred letters per week from my constituents and many more from others across the country, on a variety of issues, including epilepsy and legislation of concern to others who have disabilities.

All Congressional offices keep track of the amount of mail which encourages a Member to vote for or against a bill. All letters are answered. It is obviously crucial to generate as many letters as you can, especially if an issue is controversial, or receiving a lot of press attention. Every letter counts!

The best letters are those that are written in your own words. Always identify yourself as a parent of a child with epilepsy. Try to focus on one issue or bill. If you can, identify the bill by its name and/or number. Also try to keep to the equivalent of one typewritten page. Be as factual as you can, but don't feel that you have to be an expert on the bill. Write about how your child will be affected by specific legislation.

Be as clear as possible and state exactly what you want the legislator to do.

Although the number of letters received on an issue is important, pre-printed or form letters do not have as much impact on a Member as personal letters. I have been very impressed in my career by the quantity and quality of letters that parents of children with disabilities can generate on important issues. You would be surprised at the numbers of letters one parent can generate.

A Washington public policy analyst once told me that there is something called the "10 Factor" in disability rights advocacy—that is, there are at least ten people who are in some way connected to a child or adult who has a disability (relatives, teachers, neighbors, friends) and are willing to write a letter on an important issue to that child or adult's life. Take advantage of that!

Telegrams or overnight letters are also a useful way of communicating your message, particularly if time is short. You may send a "Public Opinion Message," which is a type of telegram specifically designed to be sent to the President, Members of Congress, and other public officials.

Phone Calls

Telephoning a Member's district or Washington office can be useful in some instances, but it will rarely put you in touch with the Member. Always identify yourself, state the title and number of the bill you are calling about, and concisely state the action you would like the Member to take on it. It is best to follow up your phone call with a letter to ensure that all of your concerns are conveyed.

Conclusion

Over the past fifteen years, parents, individuals with disabilities, and other advocates have been very effective in securing major legislative changes affecting millions of Americans with disabilities. This struggle has not been easy, and it has been fraught with setbacks and disappointments. However, perseverance pays off in the legislative process.

Remember, very few, if any, bills emerge out of the legislative process as they were initially drafted. It takes a majority of votes to win. Just because a bill is compromised or amended does not mean that you have failed. You might have lost a battle, but you have not lost the war.

I hope you find your experience with the legislative process to be as exciting and rewarding as mine has been. By working together, we can have that brighter future.

Parent Statements

I think that the new push in legislation is going to be on what happens to the kids after they turn twenty-one. There's so much that's been done for early intervention and for special education. Now they're looking beyond the school years.

Most of me is scared about the future. I'm so proud of him for being able to make it through school under the circumstances and graduate on time next year. But that big hole after graduation scares us to death.

My step-son is severely retarded and institutionalized. My husband often compares the feelings we have for our sons. Sometimes I tell him, "This may sound awful, but in a way you are lucky because you know where Gary is, where he's going." With Stephen it's so uncertain. Where will he be in five years, ten years? Will he be able to do this or that? What will be available for him? But no one knows.

What will happen to our children after they leave the protection of PL 94–142? How will their world be?

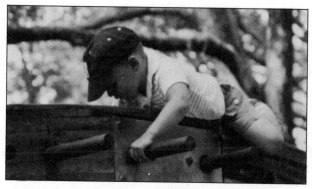

If a mere one percent of the 100,000 people diagnosed with epilepsy each year wrote their elected officials, there could be great strides in research, greater emphasis on programs such as respite care, trained day care providers, and even better educational programs.

Legislative issues that concern me right now are educational programs for handicapped kids. Every time there's a budget crunch there tends to be a desire to cut back on special education. That's where the least amount of people are probably hit so that tends to be where they're cut.

People are just coming out of the closet about epilepsy. Legislation is important if we're to go forward.

Having a handicapped child has brought to our attention the needs that are not being addressed by our society for all handicapped children and their families and the need to do something about it. We are becoming more active to help improve rights and services for the handicapped.

His superior education in special education has turned me around. I let my elected officials know how valuable it is. Otherwise they could easily cut back on special ed if no one reminds them.

Am I aware of legislative issues that affect people with epilepsy? No, should I be? How can I be? Can I really make any difference at all?

I began writing to my congressman; just dropping a line whenever something popped into my head. Do you know that from time to time his office calls to get my opinion? They really do listen.

Parents have caused most of the changes in legislation.

TEN

The Epilepsy Foundation of America

ANN SCHERER*

The Epilepsy Foundation of America (EFA) is the national organization that represents people with epilepsy and is devoted to helping create a better world for you and your children. It is the place to turn, on local and national levels, for everything from technical information to finding another parent to talk to. Among organizations dealing with special needs, the EFA's size and scope of services is unique. The following story illustrates the impact its information had on one family.

> Two years ago a Connecticut family faced a baffling medical problem. Their five-year-old daughter began to have frequent seizures affecting one side of her body. After exhaustive testing the diagnosis was Rasmussen's encephalitis, a rare, progressive brain disease about which little was known and for which there was no known effective treatment other than trying to stop the seizures. The child's brain was being destroyed from within and nothing could be done about it.
>
> The family did not give up. They tried to find out all they could about this disease. They called the Epilepsy Foundation of America's

---

* Ann Scherer is Director, Information and Education, the Epilepsy Foundation of America.

library. The librarian had nothing to tell them at the time, but took their name and address and promised to get back to them if any new research or information came along.

Several months later the librarian came across an article about a new kind of surgery to treat Rasmussen's encephalitis. She wrote to the family.

The result was that the child had the surgery and is now slowly making the long climb back to what everyone hopes will be a normal childhood without seizures.

The story you have just read shows how something as undramatic as an information service can be the vital link to a better life for someone with epilepsy.

This chapter describes how the Epilepsy Foundation of America came into existence and how parents, doctors, lawmakers, people with epilepsy, and other concerned people joined together to change how society responds to epilepsy—and epilepsy's consequences.

Forging A Movement

Ancient civilizations often regarded epilepsy—and most illness—as divine punishment for evil behavior. The psychiatrists of the late 19th and early 20th century discarded divine involvement in epilepsy but substituted the idea that epilepsy could cause evil behavior. They suggested all kinds of theories linking epilepsy to criminality, mental deterioration, uncontrollable rage, and odd personality traits. Their ideas have been *thoroughly discredited*—but their shadow remains. It lingers in out-of-date texts, in old wives' tales, and in the feelings people have somehow absorbed from an earlier age. These attitudes led to many unfair restrictions on people with epilepsy, restrictions that lasted for generations.

Even into the 1940s, people with epilepsy were forbidden to marry in some states, sterilization was permitted, and children were often barred from regular schools.

The situation improved in the late 1940s. Research led to more effective treatment and better seizure control. Groups sprang up providing a blend of services combining information and emotional support for people with epilepsy. None of them, however, had the strength or the resources to make a significant impact on the lives of people with epilepsy. Yet these groups did make some important contributions. They established or supported clinics. They raised funds to purchase EEG machines. They mounted public education campaigns to educate people. Some successfully lobbied for changes in laws, especially laws forbidding people with epilepsy to marry. The efforts of others led to the National Institute for Neurological and Communicative Disorders 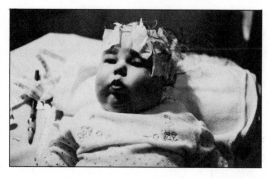 and Stroke (NINCDS). This National Institutes of Health branch is the primary source of federal research funds for epilepsy.

As time went on, people began to see that there had to be an organized public voice for epilepsy in Congress, and at state and local levels.

In 1968, after a series of mergers, the Epilepsy Foundation of America was born. Since then dramatic changes have occurred to improve the quality of life for people with seizures. For example, funds were provided for the first blood level monitoring demonstration projects. Drug level testing programs were sponsored so that there were uniform and accurate tests used in all blood labs. However, the major turning point for the epilepsy movement came later when the federal government recognized a need to examine what epilepsy was doing to people around the country and determine what society's response should be.

In 1945 Dr. William Lennox, the great American pioneer of modern epilepsy treatment, had testified in Congress in support of a Senate bill which called for "research, and investigation as to the cause, prevention, treatment and possible cure of epilepsy." He told the committee there that "of all the handicaps you and your committee are studying, epilepsy without a doubt is the least understood...and is the most neglected. Like the lepers of ancient times, epileptics still 'dwell without the city' of public understanding and philanthropy."

Despite Dr. Lennox's efforts, the bill did not pass in 1945. There was no grass roots movement, no strong lobbying effort. But in 1973, the effort was made again and this time the outcome was very different.

In response to pressure from the EFA, a bill was introduced in Congress calling for the establishment of a commission to investigate the way epilepsy was treated in the United States and make recommendations for change. It was attached to a massive health bill that was initially vetoed, but was reintroduced, and finally became law in 1975.

In July of that year, thirty years after Dr. Lennox had tried so hard to convince Congress to take action, the Secretary of the Department of Health, Education and Welfare (now Health and Human Services) appointed the Commission for the Control of Epilepsy and Its Consequences to take an official look at the problems of epilepsy.

The commission report stated that: 1) there was widespread misunderstanding and lack of information about epilepsy and 2) people with epilepsy want to be involved in their own care, and to be independent and productive.

One of the special studies the commission asked for was a detailed analysis of about twenty federal programs that might affect people with epilepsy. The outcome was a series of specific recommendations for changes to get rid of some of the barriers that limited access to government programs. It was the commission that recommended adding the word "seizures" to regulations implementing The Education for All Handicapped Children Act, Public Law 94–142, and designating epilepsy as an "underserved" group by the Rehabilitation Services Administration and "handicapped" as a target group for the old CETA program.

It also called for the prompt approval of Valproate (Depakene, Depakote) as an antiepileptic drug and urged greater efforts to make new drugs available more quickly. The EFA worked very hard to bring this issue before the press and the regulatory agencies responsible for the drug's approval. The advocacy efforts were rewarded. In 1978 the Food and Drug Administration (FDA) approved the medication for use against epilepsy, an estimated two years ahead of schedule.

At the same time the EFA was advocating for FDA approval of Valproate, Dr. Bernard Abrams, an optometrist from Columbus, Ohio, and his wife Shirley, mounted a personal crusade to get it approved in this country for their daughter, Felice, who had uncontrolled seizures. The drug had been used successfully overseas for many years for the type of seizures their daughter had, and they were determined that she – and others like her – should have the opportunity to benefit from the drug. The press gave their efforts a lot of attention. The pressure that attention generated brought other parents forward to work with the EFA and helped create a climate of public opinion in favor of approving the drug.

The commission recommended many other positive changes, including establishment of a National Information Center on Epilepsy, more research on infantile spasms, earlier recognition of seizures in high risk children, greater protection for employees with epilepsy against unfair employment practices, more education about epilepsy in the schools, a relaxation of barriers against the entry of people with epilepsy into the armed forces, greater attention to the needs of people with mental health problems in addition to epilepsy, more public education, and better health care in institutions.

The Commission for the Control of Epilepsy and Its Consequences, and the EFA, as the group carrying out many of the commission's recommendations, have made significant changes in the way our country views the disorder, even though there is still so much to be done.

One of its recommendations was the public education campaign that allows the public to see people with epilepsy as people with whom they can identify, people whom they could like and admire. The EFA responded with a television campaign featuring people with epilepsy who had achieved success in many different fields. "We're out to change your thinking about epilepsy," said Rep. Tony Coelho, of California, as it began. "People still have weird ideas about people like us," said Dr. Woody Anderson, a research physicist with the Navy. "They don't know you can play professional basketball," said 76er's player Bobby Jones, "or professional hockey," said Gary Howatt, of the New York Islanders, "or a working mom" said government employee, Sylvia Thomas, "or a normal kid," said ten-year-old Jim Shimmel, "or even a U.S. Congressman – with epilepsy," finished Rep. Coelho.

This kind of educational message, combined with dramatic advances in treatment is creating a new world for our children. Never forget that this new world is the product of many years of hard work by parents, professionals, advocates, and people with epilepsy. This long battle will not be won, however, until the last shreds of misunderstanding disappear and *all* forms of epilepsy yield to treatment.

The Epilepsy Foundation Of America Today

The EFA provides numerous services throughout the country to people with epilepsy and their families. It has developed working relationships with various federal, state, and local government units. It has established professional ties with national and international organizations.

In form it is an organization with a national, state, and local structure. Independently operated state and local groups are bound to the national organization by an affiliation agreement.

Major EFA Programs Usually Conducted At The State Or Local Level

Information and Referral Services. A core program service. It tells people where to find help and gives out basic information about epilepsy and local services, including sources of medical treatment.

School Alert. An educational program to improve the school environment for the child with epilepsy. It does so by giving teachers, school nurses, and other school personnel information about epilepsy and first aid. Information is also given to students. This is one of the most important programs in which parents can become involved.

Epilepsy Month. A program of intensive public information and education is conducted during November, National Epilepsy Month. The organization provides press and publicity materials, TV and radio messages, and conducts fund raising efforts.

Speaker's Bureau. An educational service to provide trained speakers to talk to groups and clubs about epilepsy.

Professional Education. This program ranges from a full-day training seminar for doctors, or an in-service presentation to personnel directors, or a series of lectures on seizure management for police and firemen. In the course of their work, many people come in contact with those who have epilepsy. This program is designed to help them do a better job of fulfilling their professional responsibilities.

Advocacy. Advocacy may include helping people to be more effective in dealing with red tape and bureaucracy on their own, or it may involve training a volunteer advisor to go with someone to a meeting or an interview in which the person has to make a case either for himself or his child. Advocacy sometimes involves getting experts to testify in support of better services or the establishment of some needed facility, like a group home for young adults. Basically, though, advocacy means speaking up, speaking out, and being heard—whether for yourself or on behalf of others.

Recreation. This is a broad term and it covers activities like camping for children and social activities for teenagers and adults.

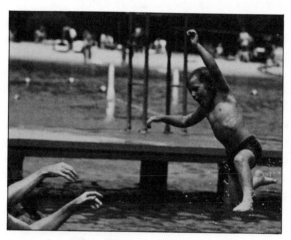

Counseling. Counseling may be offered by a staff professional or through peer-support programs involving people with epilepsy or parents.

Self-Help. The idea of gaining strength from sharing experiences has been successful for many people. Support groups for adults, teenagers, and parents are a rapidly growing part of the EFA system's program activities.

Employment Services. Most are based on the foundation's national Training and Placement Services (TAPS), a program that combines mutual support, job clubs, employer education, and follow up services after employment.

Group Homes. A few affiliates operate residence programs for adults with epilepsy who need help in day-to-day living but are not so handicapped that they need more care. The actual design of the program often depends on the source of funds, but in general they range all the way from individual apartments to group homes and day care centers. Many offer a bridge between living at home and complete independence.

EFA Programs Conducted At The National Level

Research. Each year the foundation supports a series of individual research projects which have competed against each other for funding. *Epilepsy Advances,* a quarterly newsletter for the scientific community, reports on what's new in clinical research and informs clinical researchers what's new in basic research.

Professional Education and Training. This activity sponsors educational seminars for doctors and an international visiting professor program to foster the exchange of knowledge between nations. The foundation also supports fellowships for physician-researchers and medical students. There is a growing emphasis on providing fellowships in the behavioral sciences as well.

Information and Referral. Currently, about twenty thousand telephone and mail requests for information are received every year. The number has jumped sharply since the start of a toll-free information service (1–800–EFA–1000) in 1986. Anyone who contacts the foundation by letter or phone gets a personal letter in response. Requests for technical information may be sent to the National Epilepsy Library and Resource Center (see below). Writers and callers are provided with the most up-to-date information on resources in their own areas, often as close to home as within the caller's zip code.

National Epilepsy Library and Resource Center. This is the place the family went for information about Rasmussen's encephalitis. Every year the Library and Resource Center does literature searches for doctors and other professionals and helps direct families to sources of information that may help them. The library has computer links to all the major research collections, and some affiliates are tied in to the library through their own computers.

Advocacy. This program works to represent the interests of people with epilepsy in Congress by lobbying for change and working in coalitions. Every year the foundation testifies in support of key government programs—epilepsy research, rehabilitation programs, financial aid for the disabled, better access to insurance, improved quality of medical care, respite programs, and dozens of other issues which affect the lives of people with epilepsy. The foundation also supports an active legal advocacy program. Although it cannot offer legal advice directly to individuals, it has two attorneys on staff whose job is to provide general information on legal matters, to work with attorneys and, in selected cases, to write friend of the court briefs. These briefs are statements which explain key issues in which epilepsy is involved. Occasionally, when the circumstances merit it, EFA provides limited financial assistance for case-related expenses like filing fees and similar costs. However, this is only done when the outcome of a particular lawsuit looks as if it will advance the well-being of people with epilepsy in general by establishing an important precedent or point of law.

Information and Education. The national office produces information materials for the public and for the media. It distributes about seven hundred thousand pamphlets a year, sends out television and radio messages, and sends printed advertisements to seven hundred magazines. It distributes information materials to individuals and groups, along with films, tapes, and reading lists. News releases are sent regularly to the press. The whole effort is designed to accomplish two primary goals: getting rid of outdated ideas about epilepsy and improving public understanding of what epilepsy is and how it is treated.

Employment. The Training and Placement Services (TAPS) program began in 1976 as a demonstration project to test a new way of helping people with epilepsy find jobs. The program is now placing over a thousand people with epilepsy in jobs each year.

Membership. The foundation's membership is open to all. Benefits of membership include the *National Spokesman*, the EFA newspaper, which covers research, legal issues, national developments, affiliate news, and the Congressional scene. By special arrangement with the American Association of Retired Persons (AARP), EFA members may participate in the AARP prescription pharmacy program and buy their epilepsy medications and other drug products at discount prices.

National Conference. A national conference is held each year to bring together representatives of all the affiliated organizations and others who serve people with epilepsy or who are advocates for adults and children with epilepsy.

Winning Kids Program. This program encourages self-esteem and rewards achievement in children who have epilepsy. It developed out of a national poster child contest composed of children who symbolized the potential of most children with epilepsy to live normal lives. Designed originally to change the misconception that children with epilepsy were somehow different, this program celebrates the ability of all children to win out over adversity to achieve success. Each year EFA affiliates enter children as their "Winning Kids" and one of them is chosen to represent the others as the national "winning kid."

Getting Involved

If you are the parent of a child with epilepsy, we urge you to contact your local EFA affiliate and become a part of its programs. Become a speaker at school gatherings. Get involved with parent groups.

Conclusion

Working together, we can bring about positive changes that will directly influence your child's life and the lives of hundreds of thousands of other children. We look forward to strong growth in all aspects of the organization, and especially in the parent programs. The whole organized epilepsy movement will benefit when that happens, but the ones who'll benefit most of all will be our children.

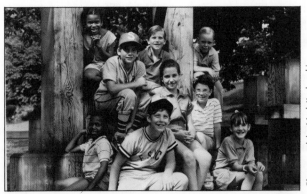

Photograph by Mark Kozlowski

GLOSSARY

Absence–New name for petit-mal seizure. Characterized by brief lapses of consciousness, usually not more than ten seconds. There may be eye blinking or twitching of the mouth associated with it. A generalized seizure.

ACTH–The acronym for Adrenocorticotropin which is the hormone excreted by the anterior pituitary gland. This steroid medication is used to treat infantile spasms and other forms of myoclonic seizures.

Acute–Sudden onset and lasting a short time.

Adaptive physical education–Physical education aimed at helping a person gain skills necessary to function in his world.

Advocacy–Supporting or promoting a cause. Speaking out.

Anticonvulsant–Drug used to control seizures. Even though all seizures are not convulsions, this term is commonly used. Antiepileptic is the preferred word, although both are acceptable.

Antiepileptic–Drug used to control seizures.

Assessment–Process to determine a child's strengths and weaknesses. Includes testing and observations performed by a team of professionals, including parents. Usually used to determine special education needs. Term is used interchangeably with evaluation.

Atonic drop–A seizure with a sudden and complete loss of muscle tone resulting in a fall. This seizure is generalized.

Attention deficit disorder–A condition that represents a child of average or above average intelligence with one or more learning disabilities. Usually is distractable and hyperactive, develops emotional and/or social problems as a result.

Attention span–The amount of time one is able to concentrate on a task. Also called "attending" in special education jargon.

Auditory–Relating to the ability to hear.

Automatism–A behavior during a seizure that looks like intentional movements: fidgeting with buttons, walking around, verbalizations, or chewing motions but is actually unintentional and the person is unaware of the movements or unable to control them.

Aura – The time just before a seizure that is like deja vu. A feeling that is the part of the seizure before unconsciousness and the person can remember it. A warning that a seizure is coming on. A "funny feeling."

Beneficiary – The person indicated in a trust or insurance policy to receive any payments that become due.

Benign – Having good outcome. Not likely to get worse; harmless.

Benign paroxysmal vertigo – A state of dizziness that is sometimes confused with a seizure. Similar to a fainting spell.

Blood Level – antiepileptic drugs are carried to the brain by the blood. Physicians determine how much medicine is in your child's body by taking a blood sample.

Carbamazepine – Tegretol. An antiepileptic. A seizure medication.

Case manager – The person responsible for taking care of coordination of school records and communication between team members.

CAT scan (CT Scan) – Computerized axial tomography. The process of taking X-ray pictures of the brain which show possible malformations.

Central nervous system – The brain and spinal cord are the receivers of sensory information, which processes and sends motor impulses to the muscles.

Cerebral palsy – Brain damage caused at birth or shortly thereafter. Affects the motor areas of the brain.

Cerebellum – Part of the brain that controls movement and equilibrium.

Cerebral cortex – Surface of the brain which also controls intellectual function, such as thinking, remembering, imagining, and movement.

Cerebrum – The biggest part of the brain, located in the upper part of the head and has three parts: frontal lobe, parietal lobe, and temporal lobe. Thinking, learning, and remembering are located in this area.

Chronic – Lasts for a long time. Doesn't go away.

Clinical – The results, or what "shows" physically. The behaviors that can be observed.

Clonazepam – Antiepileptic in the Benzodiazepine family, or Valium family. Clonopin.

Clonic – Seizure that affects the whole brain, and is muscle contractions and relaxations repeated in a series.

Clonopin – Clonazepam. An antiepileptic. A seizure medication.

Cognitive – Relating to the process of thinking. The ability to receive information, process, and analyze it.

Complex partial – Name of seizure that is located in one part of the brain, the temporal lobe, and causes loss of consciousness. Formerly called temporal lobe epilepsy or psychomotor epilepsy.

Consciousness – The state of awareness. Awake and participating.

Congenital – Something present at birth.

Convulsion – Involuntary contractions of the muscles. A seizure.

Corpus callosum – A large bundle of nerve fibers that connects the left and right cerebral hemispheres.

Cost-of-care liability – The right of a state providing care to a handicapped person to charge for the care and to collect from the handicapped person's estate.

Depakene – Valproic Acid in liquid form. An antiepileptic seizure medication.

Depakote – Valproic Acid in pill form with enteric coating that dissolves after passing through the stomach into the intestine.

Deja-vu – The feeling that "this has happened before." Sometimes precedes a seizure that is located in the temporal lobe.

Development – The process of growth and learning during which a child acquires skills and abilities.

Developmental milestone – A developmental goal that functions as a measurement of developmental progress over time.

Developmentally delayed – A person whose development is slower than normal.

Diamox – Acetazolamide. An antiepileptic seizure medication.

Diazepam–Valium. Frequently used to break cycle of seizures.

Dilantin–Phenytoin. An antiepileptic seizure medication.

Discretionary trust–A trust in which the trustee (the person responsible for governing the trust) has the authority to use or not use the trust funds for any purpose, as long as funds are expended only for the beneficiary.

Disinherit–To deprive someone of an inheritance. Parents of handicapped children may do this to prevent the state from imposing cost-of-care liability on their child's assets.

Dispute resolution procedures–The procedure established by law and regulation for the fair resolution of disputes regarding a child's special education.

Due process hearing–Part of the procedures established to protect the rights of parents and exceptional children during disputes under Public Law 94–142. These are hearings before an impartial person to review the identification, evaluation, placement, and services by a handicapped child's educational agency.

Early intervention–The specialized way of interacting with infants to minimize the effects of conditions that can delay early development.

Early development–Development during the first three years of life.

Electroencephalogram–The EEG. The machine and test to determine levels of electrical discharge from nerve cells.

Enzyme–A secretion from cells that change chemicals in other body substances.

Epilepsia partialis continua–A simple partial seizure that produces a constant jerking on one side of the body. Usually does not cause loss of consciousness.

Epilepsy–A recurrent condition caused by abnormal electrical discharges in the brain that causes seizures.

Epileptic pseudoretardation–Intellectual delay caused by the interruption of brain function due to seizures. May be reversible if seizures are controlled.

Estate planning–Formal, written arrangements for handling the possessions and assets of people after they have died.

Ethosuximide–See Zarontin.

Etiology–The study of the cause of disease.

Evaluation–See assessment.

Expressive language–The ability to use gestures, words, and written symbols to communicate.

Extension–The straightening of the muscles and limbs.

Family coordinator–The professional in the special education team responsible for the student's and family's needs, educational as well as other.

FAPE–See Free Appropriate Public Education

Febrile–fever.

Febrile seizure–Seizures that are associated with fever.

Fine motor–The use of the small muscles of the body, such as the hands, feet, fingers, and toes.

Flexion–The bending of the muscles and limbs.

Focal–One area of the brain. A seizure that begins in or remains in just one area of the brain.

Free Appropriate Public Education–The basic right to special education established under Public Law 94–142, The Education for All Handicapped Children Act.

Generalized–Refers to all the brain. A tonic/clonic or absence seizure is activity throughout all the brain.

Generalized tonic/clonic–Seizure that involves the whole brain. Formerly called grand mal seizures.

Genetic–Inherited.

Grand mal–See tonic/clonic seizure.

Gross motor–The use of the large muscles of the body.

Half life–The time it takes a drug to decrease in potency in the blood by fifty percent.

Handicapped–Refers to people who have some sort of disability, including physical disabilities, mental retardation, sensory impairments, behavioral disorders, learning disabilities, and multiple handicaps.

Hyperactivity–Specific nervous system based difficulty which makes it hard for a child to control muscle (motor) behavior.

Hyperventilation–Breathing fast and deep. Causes a feeling of faintness and in some people, seizures.

Hypotonia–Very low muscle tone.

Hypsarrythmia–The brain wave tracing associated with infantile spasms.

Identification–The determination that a child should be evaluated as a possible candidate for special education services.

Idiopathic–Without a cause. No reason. Primary epilepsy.

IEP (Individualized Education Program)–The written report that details the special education program to be provided to a child.

Infantile spasms–A type of epilepsy that occurs at about three months, or during the first year of life.

Intelligence quotient (IQ)–A measure of cognitive ability based on specifically designed standardized tests.

Interpretive–The session during which parents and teachers review and discuss the results of a child's evaluation.

Juvenile myoclonic–Age related seizure appearing in adolescence. Seizures occur in the morning and are tonic/clonic.

Intractable–Doesn't go away.

Ketogenic diet–Diet high in fat, usually four times greater than carbohydrates and protein. Sometimes is effective in the control of myoclonic seizures.

Kilogram–Metric unit of weight that is 1000 grams and equal to 2.2 pounds.

Kindling–The "learned" response of the cells in the brain to have more seizures.

Lateralization–Affecting one hemisphere of the brain.

Least restrictive environment–The requirement under Public Law 94–142 that handicapped children receiving special education must be made a part of a regular school to the fullest extent possible. Included in the law as a way of ending the traditional practice of isolating handicapped children.

Lennox Gastaut – A syndrome characterized by drop attacks, absence, tonic/clonic, tonic axial seizures with extension and complex partial. Difficult to treat.

Lesion – An injury resulting in a change in the tissue.

Local Education Agency (LEA) – The agency responsible for providing educational services on the local (city, county, and school district) level.

Luxury trusts – A trust that describes the kind of allowable expenses in a way that excludes the cost of care in state-funded programs in order to avoid cost-of-care liability.

Magnetic Resonance Image – Computerized brain scan. Very detailed.

Mainstream – The practice of involving handicapped children in regular school and preschool environments.

Mental Retardation – Below normal mental function. Children who are mentally retarded learn more slowly than other children, but "mental retardation" itself does not indicate the child's level of dysfunction. The level of mental function may not be identifiable until a much later age.

Metabolism – The biochemical changes in cells that provides energy.

Methsuximide – See Celontin.

Monotherapy – The use of a single antiepileptic. The trend in neurology is to use a single drug. Side effects are fewer even if the control of seizures remains the same.

Motor planning – The ability to think through and carry out a physical task.

Motor – The ability to move oneself.

MRI – See Magnetic Resonance Image.

Multidisciplinary – Term used to describe a group of professionals, all with different areas of expertise, working on one child's medical or educational program.

Multihandicapped – Having more than one handicap.

Muscle tone – Constant neural stimulation that keeps the muscles slightly tense.

Myoclonic – Sudden massive jerk of the muscles. Sometimes the entire body jerks, or just a limb. This seizure effects whole brain, or is generalized.

Mysoline – Primidone. An antiepileptic seizure medication.

Neonatal – The period just after birth.

Neurodevelopmental treatment (NDT) – An approach to therapy that emphasizes inhibiting abnormal patterns of posture and movement and facilitates the greatest possible variety of innate normal basic motor patterns. Used by physical, occupational, and speech therapists.

Neuron – Nerve cell in the brain.

Neurotransmitter – The chemical substance between nerve cells in the brain which transmit electrical signals.

Noncompliance – Not taking seizure medication as prescribed.

Nonconvulsive – A seizure that is not characterized by convulsive movements. An absence seizure is nonconvulsive.

Occupational therapist (OT) – A therapist who specializes in improving the development of fine motor and adaptive skills.

Oral motor – The movement of muscles in and around the mouth.

Partial seizure – The name for a focal or local seizure. Indicates that the abnormal discharge took place in one specific part of the brain.

PET Scan – See Position Emission Tomography.

Petit mal – Old name for absence seizure.

Phenobarbital – An antiepileptic. A seizure medication.

Phenytoin – See Dilantin.

Photic stimulation – A flashing strobe light is used during an EEG to determine if a seizure can be induced.

Physical therapist (PT) – A therapist who works with motor skills.

Placement – The selection of the educational program for a child who needs special education programs.

Polypharmacy – The use of two or more antiepileptics at the same time. Neurologists are steering away from using more than one antiepileptic at a time since this can cause seizures.

Position Emission Tomography – Test that identifies metabolic activity.

Primary epilepsy – The name for epilepsy that has an unknown cause. Also called idiopathic epilepsy.

Primidone – See Mysoline.

Prognosis – A prediction or forecast about the future.

Prophylactic therapy – Treatment to prevent further seizures.

Psychomotor seizure – Old term for complex partial seizure.

Protein binding – The way a drug attaches itself to a blood cell to catch a ride to the brain.

Public Law 94–142 The Education for All Handicapped Children Act of 1975 – Provides for a "free appropriate public education" for handicapped children.

Pyknoleptic petit mal – Syndrome of childhood absence seizures which is primary generalized epilepsy and is without a known cause.

Receptive language – The ability to understand spoken and written communication as well as gestures.

Rectal Diazepam – Valium administered rectally by a tube. Absorption is much faster than intramuscularly or by mouth. Often used to stop status epilepticus.

Related services – Services that enable a child to benefit from special education such as speech, occupational, and physical therapies. Transportation is also a related service.

Rolandic – Sleep related seizure associated with early years.

Screening test – A test given to groups of children to sort out those that need further evaluation.

Secondary epilepsy – Seizure with a known cause, such as a lesion or damage due to infection. Also called symptomatic epilepsy.

Seizure–Abnormal electrical discharges in nerve cells in the brain.

Self-esteem–How a person feels about himself.

Sensory–Having to do with the senses; sight, sound, touch, taste, and smell.

Sensory integration therapy–Treatment involving sensory stimulation and adaptive responses to it according to a child's neurologic need. The goal is to improve the way the brain processes and organizes sensations.

Sensory integration–The ability to process sensations like touch, smell, sound, light, and movement.

Serum blood levels–The level of antiepileptics in the blood. Used to monitor drug therapy in the control of seizures.

Simple partial–A seizure that remains in one area of the brain and consciousness is not lost.

Social Security Disability Insurance (SSDI)–A federal public assistance program for qualified disabled people.

Special needs–Needs generated by a person's handicap.

Special education–Specialized instruction based on educational disabilities determined by a team evaluation. It must be precisely matched to educational needs and adapted to the child's learning style.

Speech/language pathologist–A highly trained therapist who works to improve speech and language skills, as well as improve oral motor abilities.

Status epilepticus–Seizures that do not remit but continue either in bursts or nonstop. Tonic/clonic status is life threatening and requires emergency medical care.

Steady state–This term describes the antiepileptic drug level in the blood once it has reached a therapeutic level. Daily doses of medication maintain this level.

Stimulant–A psychotropic drug that is often used in children to control hyperactivity. (Ritalin and Dexedrine)

Subclinical–That which does not show.

Support trust–A trust that requires that funds be expended to pay for the beneficiary's expenses of living, such as housing, food, and transportation.

Symptomatic–Has a cause that is identified.

Syncopal–Short period of unconsciousness. Fainting.

Tactile defensive–An overreaction, fear of touch, or extreme dislike.

Tactile–Having to do with touch.

Tegretol–Carbamazepine. An antiepileptic seizure medication.

Temporal lobe–Section of the brain located on the top front. Contains auditory, language, speech, and behavioral receptive areas.

Temporal lobe epilepsy–Old term for complex partial seizures. Also used to be called psychomotor epilepsy.

The Education for All Handicapped Children Act of 1975 (EAHCA) Public Law 94–142–See Public Law 94–142.

Therapeutic blood level–Each antiepileptic drug has a level at which it is most effective. A drug is taken, slowly absorbed and with each dose, a level is maintained that provides the most effective protection against seizures.

Tonic–Seizure that is a stiffening of the body. Affects the whole brain.

Tonic/clonic–New term for grand mal seizure. A seizure that effects the whole brain. A convulsive seizure and one most people associate with epilepsy.

Trimethadione–An antiepileptic seizure medication.

Trunk rotation–The ability to turn and twist the trunk. Necessary skill for walking.

Valproate (Valproic Acid)–See Depakote, Depakene.

Vestibular system or input–The sensory system that responds to the position of the head in relation to gravity and movement. Input means activities like bouncing on a ball, or swinging on a hammock.

Visual motor–The skill required to carry out a task such as putting a puzzle piece into the puzzle or a key into a keyhole.

Vocational training–Training for a job. Learning skills to perform in the work place.

Zarontin–Ethosuximide. An antiepileptic seizure medication.

CLASSIFICATION OF SEIZURES

It is wise for parents and professionals to become familiar with both the old and the new terminology for seizures. Due to recent research, there have been great advances in understanding the central nervous system. Scientists continue to unravel the mystery of the brain and, along with it, the mystery of epilepsy. One of the results of progress is that new seizure types are discovered and named. In the old days, seizures were commonly referred to as "little seizures" (petit mal) and "big seizures" (grand mal). Today, we can use clinical observations (what we see) as well as many sophisticated tests and machines, to locate exact areas in the brain where abnormal electrical discharges occur. And, terminology will change to keep pace with those discoveries.

Understanding the evolution of the research and terminology of epilepsy will help you to explain your child's condition to others. You may find that teachers, school nurses, pediatricians, and other medical professionals—because they are not directly involved with epilepsy—have not kept up with the research. Not only do they need to learn the new terms, but they also need to learn about the new drugs and proper first aid. In addition, it is also vital—and cannot be stressed enough—that what you see when your child has a seizure is critical to accurate diagnosis. That is why it is vital for you to feel at ease using the terminology of epilepsy when you are discussing your child's condition. The following chart shows the current and the former terminology.

CURRENT TERM

PARTIAL SEIZURES

simple partial	focal motor, focal sensory, Jacksonian
complex partial	psychomotor, temporal lobe
partial seizure, secondarily generalized	focal and grand mal convulsion

GENERALIZED SEIZURES

tonic-clonic	grand mal
absence	petit mal
atonic seizure	drop attack
myoclonic seizure	minor motor
infantile spasms	jackknife, salaam, or West syndrome

READING LIST

Chapters 1 and 2

Commission for the Control of Epilepsy and Its Consequences, National Institutes of Health. *Plan for Nationwide Action of Epilepsy,* Vol. 1. National Institute of Neurological and Communicative Disorders and Strokes, NIH, 1977. Once you get a grip on your child's epilepsy, you might be ready to learn about the way the epilepsy movement came about and who were the movers and shakers. This volume is a summary of the reports and research made by the commission. This report has been a critical step toward the advances in the management, research, and a national plan to prevent and control epilepsy. A highly recommended, very interesting report. Available from National Technical Information Service, Springfield, VA 22164. Ask for Ref #PB811020907. Cost is $24.95 plus $3.00 shipping and handling. You might try to find it at your local EFA affiliate or special needs library. If they don't have a copy, ask them to order one.

Dreifuss, Fritz E. *Pediatric Epileptology: Classification and Management of Seizures in the Child.* Littleton, MA: John Wright PSG, 1983. This book is a very in-depth, readable, technical textbook. It explains everything there is to know about epilepsy, seizure classifications, diagnosis, drugs, side effects, the EEG, etc. An excellent chapter on the psychosocial aspects of epilepsy finishes off a book just loaded with references for further research. Highly recommended but hard to come by. Try asking your library to make an inter-library loan from a medical school library. It takes time but well worth the wait (or buy it directly from the publisher).

Epilepsy Foundation of America. *National Spokesman.* This is the newsletter of the Epilepsy Foundation. There is not one other source of information for families as comprehensive and interesting as this. Articles range from legislative updates to how families cope. This is a must for all parents of children with epilepsy. Available from EFA at 4351 Garden City Dr., Landover, MD 20785.

Gadow, Kenneth D. *Children on Medication Volume II. Epilepsy, Emotional Disturbance, and Adolescent Disorders.* San Diego, CA, College Hill Press, 1986. Available from Council for Exceptional Children, 1920 Association Drive, Reston, VA. 22091. An excellent resource describing epilepsy, drug side effects, learning and behavior changes. A thorough, readable, and valuable resource for parents trying to identify and follow up on medication side effects. Very highly recommended and practically the only one of its kind.

Jan, James E., Robert G. Ziegler and Guiseppe Erba. *Does Your Child Have Epilepsy?* Baltimore: University Park Press, 1983. This book addresses issues about epilepsy that concern the family and the authors advocate developing a partnership with the neurologist. Recommended. Comprehensive.

Laidlaw, Mary V. and John Laidlaw. *Epilepsy Explained*. New York: Churchill Livingstone, 1984. A short book written for people who have epilepsy.

Laidlaw, Mary V. and John Laidlaw. *People with Epilepsy: How They Can be Helped*. New York: Churchill Livingstone, 1984. Is written for all those whose work involves helping people with epilepsy – GP's, nurses, social workers, teachers, clergymen, etc. Also useful for families.

Middleton, Allen H., Arthur A. Attwell and Gregory O. Walsh. *Epilepsy: A Handbook for Patients, Parents, Families, Teachers, Health and Social Workers*. Boston: Little Brown & Co., 1981. This handbook is organized by subject area in a question and answer format.

National Institutes of Health. *Epilepsy*. Medicine for the Layman series, produced by the Clinical Center Office of Clinical Reports and Inquiries (NIH, Bethesda, Md. 20205), 1982. This booklet is a succinct, factual guide to epilepsy and also answers some commonly asked questions about the condition. Simple, easy, and great to have around to hand out to friends.

O'Donohue, Niall V. *Epilepsies of Childhood*. London: Butterworths, 1985. This book is written by a professor of pediatrics at Trinity College in Dublin, Ireland. It is another textbook that is very readable and will provide answers to questions about side effects of medications. It is jammed with information and references. This book offers a glimpse into the foreign perspective regarding epilepsy today and historically. Again, you'll have to do some creative library work to get a copy, but it's well worth the effort. Be sure to get the second edition, 1985, rather than the previous printing in 1981.

Penry, J. Kiffin. *Diagnosis, Management and Quality of Life*. New York: Raven Press, 1986. This is a fine 42 page book which represents the material presented at a recent 1985 symposium of the same name. It doesn't claim to be exhaustive, rather it presents recent advances in the diagnosis and management of epilepsy.

Schumacher, Nancy Carlisle. *Epilepsy, A Personal Approach*. Cambridge, Mass: Schenkman Publishing Co., Inc., 1985. This little book approaches life from the perspective of having epilepsy. Its subjects range from treatment to advocacy.

Schneider, Joseph W. and Peter Conrad. *Having Epilepsy: The Experience and Control of Illness*. Philadelphia: Temple University Press, 1983. This is a book based on interview data from eighty people.

Sugarman, Gerald I. *Epilepsy Handbook: A Guide to Understanding Seizure Disorders.* St Louis, Missouri: C.V. Mosby Company, 1984. This is a question/answer format guide. Also has answers to questions you didn't know existed. Recommended.

Svoboda, William B. *Learning About Epilepsy.* Baltimore, MD: University Park Press, 1979. Comprehensive book that can be used by medical professionals and families alike. There is a chapter on learning disabilities as well as psychosocial issues. Recommended.

Chapter 3

Buscaglila, Leo. *The Disabled and Their Parents: A Counselling Challenge.* Thorofare, NJ: Slack, Inc., 1983. Collection of articles written by professional counselors and experienced lay people dealing with the responsibility and role of family, legal rights of handicapped persons, and counseling of disabled people and their families.

Byars, Betsy. *The Summer of the Swans.* New York: Viking Press, 1970. The story of a retarded boy and his adolescent sister. A good story for teenagers coping with a disabled sibling.

Eisenberg, M.G., L.F. Sutking, L.F. and M.A. Jansen. *Chronic Illness and Disability Through the Life Span: Effects on Self and Family.* Vol. 4. New York: Springer Publishing, 1984. Passing through the stages of life with reviews of available research. Information is based on actual clinical experiences. Successful coping techniques are included.

Hermes, Patricia. *What if They Knew.* New York: Harcourt, 1980. Ten-year-old Jeremy has epilepsy and fears that his secret will be discovered. Realistic novel is a sensitive introduction to the personal anguish of physical disabilities.

Lechtenberg, Richard. *Epilepsy and the Family.* Cambridge, MA: Harvard University Press, 1984. This book is written for families who have a member with epilepsy. It covers subjects ranging from developmental issues of the child to marital relationship of the parents.

Lickona, Thomas. *Raising Good Children.* New York: Bantam, 1983. How to help your child develop a lifelong sense of honesty, decency, and respect for others.

McCollum, Audrey. *The Chronically Ill Child: A Guide for Parents and Professionals.* Boston: Little Brown & Co., 1981. Sensitively and thoroughly covers the problems and reactions of disabled children of various age periods and of the parents who are trying to help them.

Melton, David. *Promises to Keep: A Handbook for Parents of Learning Disabled, Brain-Injured and Other Exceptional Children*. New York: Franklin Watts, 1984. A good general guide to raising and caring for special needs children.

Meyer, Donald J., Patricia Vadasy and Rebecca R. Fewell. *Living with a Brother or Sister with Special Needs*. Seattle: University of Washington Press, 1985. This book is written in common sense language that explains the various disabilities and what it feels like to live with a sibling who is handicapped.

Miezio, Peggy Muller. *Parenting Children with Disabilities*. New York: Marcel Dekker, 1983. This book is about parenting a child with special needs. It covers all stages of development, including issues of adolescence and sexuality.

Powell, Thomas H. and Peggy Ahrenhold Ogle. *Brothers & Sisters: A Special Part of Exceptional Families*. Baltimore: Paul H. Brookes Publishing Co., 1985. Comprehensive book covering all aspects of parenting as well as offering advice to professionals. Extensive reading list for siblings arranged by disabilities and age levels.

Schenk, Quentin and Emmy Lou Schenk. *Pulling up Roots*. Englewood Cliffs, NJ: Prentice Hall, 1978. Written for parents as a guide to coping with normal children not quite adolescent and not quite adult. Would be good for parents with older special needs children.

Summers, Jean Ann. *The Right to Grow Up – An Introduction to Adults with Developmental Disabilities*. Baltimore, Maryland: Paul H. Brookes Publishing Co. 1985. Book that covers what happens to the disabled child as he approaches adulthood. Parents usually focus on needs of younger children. This focuses on meeting needs to encourage independence.

Travis, G. *Chronic Illness in Children: Its Impact on Child and Family*. Stanford, CA: Stanford University Press. 1976. How a family copes with a disabled, chronically ill member. Includes the psychosocial and medical realities families face with information on coping.

Chapter 4

Association for the Care of Children's Health. *Organizing and Maintaining Support Groups for Parents of Children with Chronic Illness and Handicapping Conditions*. Washington, D.C.: ACCH (3615 Wisconsin Avenue NW, Washington, D.C. 20016), 1986. A handbook for parents and professionals forming and working in support groups. Sections address getting started, organizing, structuring and maintaining. In loose leaf format. 102 pages.

Association for the Care of Children's Health. *Parent Resource Directory.* This directory is for parents and professionals who want to talk to other parents. The listings are by state and within each state, by disability. Cross referenced in the back of the book so you can easily find parents of kids with epilepsy by looking up seizures or epilepsy. A valuable resource.

Featherstone, Helen. *A Difference in the Family: Living with a Disabled Child.* New York: Penguin, 1980. A compassionate look into the emotions of having a disabled child, based on the author's experiences and interviews with parents and professionals. Highly recommended.

Fensterheim, Herbert and Jean Baer. *Don't Say Yes When You Want To Say No.* New York: Dell Publishing, 1975. Describes hidden rules of social interaction and discusses how to get your own way without being aggressive.

Epilepsy Association of Western Washington. *My Full Life.* 8511 15th St. NE, Seattle, WA 98125. A coloring book for children with disabilities. A 43 page booklet with cheerful illustrations ranging from taking medications and eating properly to making friends.

Girion, B. *A Handful of Stars.* New York: Charles Scribner & Sons, 1981. Story of a teenage girl with epilepsy and how she copes with herself, friends, family, and school.

McCleary, Elliott H. *Your Child Has a Future.* National Easter Seal Society, 2023 West Ogden Ave., Chicago, IL 60612. A brief discussion about parenting children with disabilities, dealing with feelings, the diagnosis, family life, available help, treatment plans, and the child's rights and opportunities.

Murphy, Albert T. *Special Children, Special Parents: Personal Issues with Handicapped Children.* Englewood Cliffs, NJ: Prentice-Hall, 1981. A look into the emotions of parents of handicapped children, written with numerous statements by parents.

Perske, Robert. *Hope for Families: New Directions for Parents of Persons with Retardation or Other Disabilities.* Nashville: Abington Press, 1981. A compassionate and philosophical book for parents about adjusting to a handicapped child.

Scheiber, Barbara and Moore, Cory. *Practical Advice for Parents.* A Guide to Finding Help for Children With Handicaps. Available from Montgomery County Association for Retarded Citizens, 11600 Nebel St., Rockville, MD 20852, 1981. This booklet is a must for all families. Compassionate and thorough. Write for it.

Schleifer, Maxwell J. and Stanley D. Klein. *The Disabled Child and The Family: An Exceptional Parent Reader.* Boston: The Exceptional Parent Press, 1985. A collection of articles from *Exceptional Parent* magazine covering a wide range of topics related to having a special needs person in the family.

Simons, Robin. *After the Tears: Parents Talk about Raising a Child with a Disability.* San Diego: Harcourt Brace & Jovanovich, 1987. This is a story about many parents who have grown in the years with their disabled children and describes the stages of acceptance.

Thompson, Charlotte E. *Raising a Handicapped Child.* New York: William B. Morrow, 1986. A comprehensive guide written by a doctor who's been practicing for 30 years. Ranges from coping with the diagnosis to having fun.

Turnbull, H. Rutherford and Ann P. Turnbull. *Parents Speak Out: Then and Now.* Columbus, Ohio: Charles E. Merrill Publishing Co., 1985. A collection of articles by parents describing their experience coping with a special needs child. This second edition presents an update from parents, giving a picture of life then and now.

Wentworth, Elsie H. *Listen to Your Heart: A Message to Parents of Handicapped Children.* Boston: Houghton Mifflin, 1974. A personal book about the emotions of adjusting to a special needs child.

Chapter 5

Biller, Ernest F. *Understanding and Guiding the Career Development of Adolescents and Young Adults with Learning Disabilities.* Springfield, IL: Charles C. Thomas, 1985. This manual of career development for the learning disabled describes a model for classifying learning disabilities, the effect on career development of behaviors associated with learning disabilities, the poor career adjustment of many LD adults, and a career development curriculum that accentuates self-esteem.

Brazelton, T. Berry, M.D. *To Listen to a Child: Understanding the Normal Problems of Growing Up.* Reading, MA: Addison-Wesley Publishing Co., 1984. A guide to handling common problems encountered in childhood and adolescence.

Burns, David. *Feeling Good.* New York: NAL Penguin, Inc., 1980. Dr. Burns is a well-known psychiatrist who has helped pioneer the treatment of depression through cognitive therapy. This book presents basic ideas and offers an array of practical techniques and exercises for improving mood and one's general state of well-being. Particularly helpful for parents who may be struggling with depression.

Burns, David. *Intimate Connections*. New York: NAL Penguin, Inc., 1985. Another excellent book from Dr. Burns. This volume describes how the basic ideas of cognitive therapy are useful for solving relationship problems. The first several chapters relating to self-esteem are strongly recommended to all parents.

Campbell, Ross. *How to Really Love Your Child*. Wheaton, Illinois: Victor Books, 1984. This book, written by a child psychiatrist, provides many useful suggestions for clearly communicating unconditional love to a child. Dr. Campbell explains how to use eye contact, physical contact, focused attention, and loving discipline to give a child the message that he is loved and prized. There is a separate chapter on children with special problems, which may be of particular interest to readers of this book. While the religious orientation of the book will be irrelevant to some, most parents should find this book to be a sensitive and succinct guide to child-rearing.

Campbell, Ross. *How To Really Love Your Teenager*. Wheaton, Illinois: Victor Books, 1986. This book covers similar territory as *How To Really Love Your Child*. However, topics of particular importance to raising teenagers are effectively dealt with, such as teenage anger, adolescent depression, parental self-control, and the transition for the teenager from parent control to self-control.

Canter, Lee. *Assertive Discipline for Parents*. Santa Monica, CA: Canter and Associates, 1985. This is a fine book for parents who are struggling with discipline. The forum that is presented allows a parent to regain authority without having to resort to yelling or threats. Principles of asserted discipline have been used very effectively in classrooms throughout the country and are also highly applicable to parents. Of particular help will be the large "menu" of possible consequences, positive and negative, for children's behavior.

Clemes, Harris and Bean, Reynold. *How To Raise Teenagers' Self-Esteem*. Los Angeles, CA: Enrich/Price-Stern-Sloan, Inc., 1985. In this slender volume, the authors explain the importance of focusing on self-esteem and then define what they consider to be the four conditions that must be met for high self-esteem. Many good suggestions are offered for helping children feel connected to their family and culture, experience and appreciate their own uniqueness, grow in a sense of power and competence, and utilize models for personal development.

Corkille-Briggs, Dorothy. *Your Child's Self-Esteem*. Garden City, New York: Dalton Books, 1975. The author of this superb book explains in great detail how to help children develop the two main convictions of self-esteem that they are lovable and worthwhile. Considerable attention is given to developing adult self-esteem and to discipline. The reader may find much useful information regarding emotional aspects of child development as well.

Corkille-Briggs, Dorothy. *Celebrate Your Life*. Garden City, NY: Doubleday, 1977. This is a very readable and practical book for adults who want to give up self-critical and self-defeating emotional and behavioral patterns.

Cragg, Sheila. *Run Patty Run*. San Francisco, California: Harper and Row, 1980. Story of a teenager with epilepsy who completed a cross-country marathon at age sixteen.

Cummings, Rhoda W. and Cleborne D. Maddux. *Parenting the Learning Disabled: A Realistic Approach*. Springfield, IL: Charles C. Thomas, 1985. This book looks at the nature of learning disabilities, the effects on children as they mature, and considerations in planning for their adulthood.

Dreikurs, Rudolf. *Children: The Challenge*. New York: Hawthorn/Dutton, 1964. This well known book explains how to encourage children to develop a strong sense of personal responsibility, autonomy, and courage. The focus is consistently on developing high self-esteem in children by treating them with consideration and respect. Dr. Dreikurs and Ms. Soltz also present a very powerful approach to discipline which minimizes the use of punishment. Chapters on resisting feeling sorry for children, stimulating independence, refraining from over-protection, and the family council may be of particular interest to parents of children with epilepsy.

Dyer, Wayne. *Your Erroneous Zones*. New York: Avon Books, 1976. This was Dr. Dyer's first best-selling book which presented the radical idea that anyone can learn to be happy by identifying and eliminating their erroneous zones. Parents should benefit from this book, especially in the early chapters on self-esteem and taking responsibility for one's feelings.

Faber, Adele and Mazlish, Elaine. *How To Talk So Kids Will Listen and Listen So Kids Will Talk*. New York: Avon Books, 1980. This book provides an excellent introduction to "active listening," a very powerful means by which parents can effectively communicate with their children. The authors also offer some of the best available advice on engaging cooperation from children (without demanding, threatening, or begging), alternatives to punishment, and developing a child's autonomy. This book is easy to read and highly recommended.

Good, Julia Darnell and Joyce Good Reis. *A Special Kind of Parenting*. La Leche League, P.O. Box 1209 Franklin Park, IL 60131-8209. Covers birth to teen years. Personalized accounts include family adjustments and strengthening marriage. For parents; written by the mom of two special needs children.

Hauck, Paul. *The Rational Management of Children*. New York: Libra Publishers, 1967. Dr. Hauck presents the basic principles of rational, emotive therapy. This book will help parents learn to be less upset about their children's problems, learn how to teach their children to be emotionally responsible, and will also provide good suggestions regarding discipline.

Ilg, Frances, Louise Ames and Sidney Baker. *Child Behavior.* New York: Barnes & Noble Books, 1982. Behavior as a function of structure. The treatment of undesirable, uncomfortable, and unhealthy behavior, and how to prevent it.

Jones, Reginald L. *Reflections on Growing Up Disabled.* Council for Exceptional Children (1920 Association Drive, Reston, VA 22091), 1983. Each chapter is written by a different person who shares the childhood feelings, insights, and self-perceptions of growing up disabled. Frustrations related to learning and socialization are expressed as well as the parental view and peer misconceptions.

Kaufman, Barry Neil. *To Love Is To Be Happy With.* New York: Ballantine Books, 1977. The author is best known for his apparently miraculous work with his autistic son described in the book *Son Rise.* This book outlines the Option Method, a Socratic dialogue process designed to enable people to uncover the beliefs which contribute to undesirable emotions and behavior. The book emphasizes the importance of accepting life as it is, and of people accepting themselves. This book is strongly recommended to parents as it offers a method for coming to an increasingly accepting and peaceful position regarding having a child with medical or developmental difficulties.

Kornfield, Elizabeth J. *Dreams Come True.* Boise ID: Mountain States Press, 1986. The story of a young girl who overcame her negative feelings about having epilepsy and went on to skate. Full of photos as she was growing up and interspersed throughout the story are facts about epilepsy.

Kushner, H.S. *When Bad Things Happen to Good People.* New York: Avon, 1981. Story of a clergyman's son who died. Describes feelings, how to accept reality, and the stages of that process. Very moving.

McDaniel, Sandy and Bielen, Peggy. *Project Self-Esteem.* Rolling Hills Estates, CA: B.L. Winch and Associates, 1986. This book presents a curriculum for self-esteem development which can be used in the classroom for elementary school age children. Parents who want to see more attention to self-esteem given in their child's educational program are encouraged to consult this book and to share it with teachers and program administrators.

Perske, Robert. *New Life in the Neighborhood: How Persons with Retardation or Other Disabilities Can Help Make a Good Community Better.* Nashville: Abingdon Press, 1980. A compassionate and philosophical look at handicapped people in the community, beautifully illustrated.

Taylor, John F. *The Hyperactive Child and the Family.* (Chapter 5), New York: Dodd, Mead and Co., 1980. While this book primarily addresses hyperactivity, the chapter on self-esteem and discipline would probably be of interest and help to parents of most children with special needs. Dr. Harris helps to clarify thoughts and attitudes which hyperactive children have about themselves, and many of these are undoubtedly shared by others with special needs.

Turecki, Stanley. *The Difficult Child.* New York, Bantam Books, 1985. This is an extraordinarily helpful book for parents whose children seem to be difficult and demanding from the time they were born. Dr. Turecki and Ms. Tonner explain how research has deepened our understanding of "built in" personality differences in children, and particularly those differences which make some children easy to love and care for and others more difficult. Chapters on regaining adult authority, managing temperament, and rebuilding the family will be particularly beneficial to parents who are struggling with their children.

Wright, Logan. *Parent Power: A Guide to Responsible Childrearing.* New York: William B. Morrow & Co., 1980. Written by a child psychologist. This book focuses on discipline.

Chapter 6

Ames, Louise and Frances Ilg. *Your Three Year Old.* New York: Dell, 1981. Practical advice and enlightening psychological insights into the behavior, problems, and pleasures of the three year old.

Ames, Louise and Frances Ilg. *Your Four Year Old.* New York: Dell, 1976. Practical advice and enlightening psychological insights into the behavior, problems, and pleasures of the four year old.

Ames, Louise and Frances Ilg. *Your Five Year Old.* New York: Dell, 1979. Practical advice and enlightening psychological insights into the behavior, problems, and pleasures of the five year old.

Ames, Louise and Frances Ilg. *Your Six Year Old.* New York: Dell, 1979. Practical advice and enlightening psychological insights into the behavior, problems, and pleasure of the six year old.

Boehm, A.E. and M.A. White. *The Parents' Handbook on School Testing.* New York:Teachers College Press, 1982. Excellent guide to tests used in schools. Addresses making sense of the results and what questions parents should ask.

Brazelton, T. Berry, M.D. *Infants and Mothers: Differences in Development*. Rev. Ed. New York: Dell Publishing Co., 1983. Written by a prominent pediatrician, this book compares the development of different children during the first year of life.

Coling, Marcia Cain. *Psychological Assessment of Handicapped Children: A Guide for Parents*. Association for Retarded Citizens of Northern Virginia, 100 North Washington Street, Suite 238, Falls Church, VA 22046. This booklet is a concise, very helpful guide to the evaluation process.

Dickman, Irving and Sol Gordon. *One Miracle at a Time, How to Get Help for Your Disabled Child: From the Experience of Other Parents*. New York: Simon and Schuster, 1985. Thoughtful compilation of techniques from parents.

Green, Lawrence. *Kids Who Hate School: A Survival Handbook on Learning Disabilities*. Atlanta, Georgia: Humanics Limited, 1983. This guide for parents of learning disabled children uses case studies, anecdotal material, and educational data to tell parents how to recognize the symptoms of a learning problem and what steps to take to see if their child receives the remediation he or she needs.

Greenspan, Stanley and Nancy Greenspan. *First Feelings*. New York: Viking Penguin, 1985. Describes the steps by which a baby grows from a self-centered bundle of sensation into a feeling, caring, responsive human being. Includes milestones of a child's emotional development.

Leach, Penelope. *Your Baby and Child: From Birth to Age Five*. New York: Alfred A. Knopf, 1981. A good general parents' guide which includes all areas of health and daily care.

National Easter Seal Society. *Parents: Do You Know the Early Warning Signs of Children with Special Needs?* 2023 West Ogden Ave., Chicago, IL 60612. Early warning signs of conditions that may be disabling.

Pearlman, Laura and Kathleen Scott. *Raising the Handicapped Child*. Englewood Cliffs, NJ: Prentice-Hall, 1981. A general guide to raising handicapped children from birth to adulthood.

Prensky, Arthur L. and Helen Stein Palkes. *Care of the Neurologically Handicapped Child: A Book for Parents and Professionals*. New York: Oxford University Press, 1982. A comprehensive, yet clinical review of the treatment of neurologically handicapped children. Includes a review of professional services.

Roiphe, Herman and Anne Roiphe. *Your Child's Mind*. New York: St. Martin's/Marek, 1985. Covers every aspect of your child's mental growth. Discusses normal emotional problems and behavior common to all children, then the abnormal symptoms and patterns which are the danger signals that your child may be in difficulty.

Showalter, J. and W. Anyan. *The Family Handbook of Adolescence: A Medically Oriented Guide to the Years from Puberty to Adulthood*. Association for the Care of Children's Health, 3615 Wisconsin Avenue NW, Washington, D.C. 20016. Details common physical and psychological problems of adolescence and provides advice on care and treatment.

Smith, Sally L. *No Easy Answers: The Learning Disabled Child at Home and at School*. New York: Bantam, 1981. Recommended by the parent of a seven-year-old learning disabled child. She uses it as a step by step guide. Highly recommended.

Spitainik, Deborah M. and Irving Rosenstein. *All Children Grow and Learn: Activities for Parents of Children with Developmental Problems*. Temple University Developmental Disabilities Center, Ritter Annex, Philadelphia, PA 19122, 1976. Simple and clear explanations of developmental delays and activities to help children learn daily living skills.

Sternlich, Manny, Ph.D. and Abraham Hurwitz. *Games Children Play*. New York: Van Nostrand Reinhold, 1981. Play activities for special needs children, geared to older children or children able to communicate.

White, Burton L. *The First Three Years of Life*. Rev. ed. New York: Prentice Hall Press, 1985. One of the classics of child development.

Chapter 7

Association for Retarded Citizens. *The Partnership: How to Make it Work*. Arlington, Texas: Association for Retarded Citizens National Research and Demonstration Institute, 1977. A short pamphlet about the relationship between parents and professionals.

Atack, Sally M. *Art Activities for the Handicapped*. Englewood Cliffs, NJ: Prentice-Hall, 1982. A practical guide to creative art activities for children with learning disabilities.

Baker, Bruce L., Alan J. Brightman, et al. *Steps to Independence: A Skills Training Series for Children with Special Needs*. Champaign, IL: Research Press (2612 North Mattis, Champaign, IL 61820). The series includes eight manuals and a training guide for use by parents in the home.

Buist, Charlotte A. and Jerome L. Schulman. *Toys and Games for Educationally Handicapped Children*. Springfield, IL: Charles C. Thomas, 1976. Description of toys and games suitable for home use, arranged by sex and age interest. Focus on fine or gross motor skills, auditory perception, etc.

Children's Defense Fund. *Your Child's School Records*. 122 C St., NW, Washington, DC, 1986. An easy to use guide to your legal right to see, correct, and control access to school records yours and your children's.

Children's Defense Fund. *94–142 and 504: Numbers That Add Up to Educational Rights for Handicapped Children. A Valuable Guide for Parents and Advocates*. 122 C St. NW, Washington, DC 20001, 1984. This valuable guide is available in English and Spanish. It explains Public Law 94–142, the Education for All Handicapped Children Act and Section 504 of the Rehabilitation Act. It guides parents through the responsibilities their school districts have to any child who needs special education.

DeVilliers, Peter A. and Jill G. DeVilliers. *Early Language*. Cambridge, MA: Harvard University Press, 1979. A book describing how a child learns to communicate verbally.

From School To Working Life: Resources and Services. National Library Service for the Blind and Physically Handicapped, 1985. Provides current, practical information to facilitate the transition of disabled students to higher education or directly to work.

Goldberg, Sally. *Teaching with Toys: Making Your Own Educational Toys*. Ann Arbor, Michigan: The University of Michigan Press, 1981. A handbook for making and playing with educational toys.

Gordon, Ira. J., Barry Guinagh and R. Emile Jester. *Child Learning Through Child Play: Learning Activities for Two and Three Year Olds*. New York: St Martin's Press, 1972. A basic activity book for young children.

Gottesman, D.M. *The Powerful Parent: A Child Advocacy Handbook*. Norwalk, CT: Appleton-Century-Crofts, 1982. Advice on how to obtain educational, medical, psychological, and legal services for your child.

Grabow, Beverly W. *Your Child Has a Learning Disability – What Is It?* Chicago: National Easter Seal Society (2023 West Ogden Ave. Chicago, IL 60612), 1978. A guide for parents and classroom teachers giving encouragement that a child with a learning disability can become a self-sufficient adult through understanding, encouragement, firmness, and proper education training.

Hart, V. *Mainstreaming Children with Special Needs*. New York: Longman, 1980. Provides information about a wide range of disabilities and educational implications.

Houghton, Janaye Matteson. *Homespun Language*. New Richmond, WI: Whitehaven Publishing Co., 1982. A book of practical language lessons based on the objects and concepts of a child's daily routine. Aimed at children over two years old.

Jeffree, Dorothy and Margaret Skeffington. *Reading is for Everyone: A Guide for Parents and Teachers of Exceptional Children*. Englewood Cliffs, NJ: Prentice-Hall, 1984. Designed for parents and teachers, this book presents practical information on helping children (from normal preschoolers to students with moderate learning difficulties) learn to read.

Kames, Marie B. *Creative Games for Learning*. Reston, VA: Council for Exceptional Children (1920 Association Drive, Reston, VA 22091). Games for parents and teachers to make for young children ages 3–8.

Long, Kate. *Parents Becoming Teachers: Working with Your Handicapped Child*. Second edition. Jan Nash Valley Community Mental Health Center (301 Scott Avenue, Morgantown, WV 36505), 1981. Easy to read, illustrated with cartoons, teaches parents how to stimulate desirable and eliminate undesirable behavior in young children.

Millman, Joan and Polly Behrman. *Parents As Playmates: A Games Approach to the Pre-School Years*. New York: Human Sciences Press, 1979. A creative book of parent-child activities based on everyday life.

Morgan, D.P. *A Primer on Individualized Education Programs for Exceptional Children*. Reston, VA: Council for Exceptional Children, 1981. This book looks at developing an IEP and reveals complexities and potential obstacles. Provides very useful data, lists, figures, sample IEPs.

Shore, Kenneth. *The Special Education Handbook*. New York: Teachers College Press, 1986. Excellent and comprehensive book written for parents by a school psychologist. Really explains the special education process clearly. Highly recommended.

Thain, Wilbur S., M.D., Glendon Castio, Ph.D. and Adrienne Peterson, R.P.T. *Normal and Handicapped Children: A Growth and Development Primer for Parents and Professionals*. Littleton, MA: PSG Publishing Co., 1980. A comprehensive review of development.

Unlocking Doors. 64 page booklet designed for parents of children who benefit from Public Law 94–142. Designed to help parents communicate their needs to educators, secure rights. PACER Center Inc. 4826 Chicago Ave. South, Minn. Minn. 55417-1055.

Winton, P.J., A.P. Turnbull, J. Blacher. *Selecting a Preschool: A Guide for Parents of Handicapped Children*. Austin, Texas: Pro-Ed., 1984. Practical book for parents that provides information on how to select a preschool for their special needs child. Information on the IEP, legal rights, and strategies for monitoring.

Wilson, Nancy O. *Parents' Guide to "Teacherese": A Glossary of Special Education Terms*. Special Child Publications, 4535 Union Bay Place NE, Seattle, WA 98105. A reference defining terms.

Chapter 8

Anderson, Winifred, Stephen Chitwood, and Deidre Hayden. *Negotiating the Special Education Maze: A Guide for Parents and Teachers*. Rockville, MD: Woodbine House, 1990. A guide to helping parents get the best special education for their child through advocacy.

Apolloni, Tony and Thomas P. Cooke. *A New Look at Guardianship: Protective Services That Support Personalized Living*. Baltimore: Paul H. Brookes Publishing Co., 1984. This book reviews the options for providing future support for handicapped persons.

ARC National Insurance And Benefits Committee. *How to Provide for Their Future*. Arlington, Texas: Association For Retarded Citizens, 1984. A booklet that explains many of the concerns about wills, estate planning, insurance, and government benefits for parents of retarded children.

Bateman, B. *So You're Going to a Hearing: Preparing for Public Law 94–142 Due Process Hearing*. Northbrook, IL: Hubbard, 1980. Compact and information filled guide describes practical strategies for preparing for and taking part in the hearing.

Biklen, Douglas. *Let Our Children Go: An Organizing Manual for Advocates and Parents*. Syracuse, NY: Human Policy Press, 1979. A handbook for organizing a grassroots campaign to improve the treatment and education of exceptional children.

Budoff, Milton and Alan Orenstein. *Due Process in Special Education: On Going to a Hearing*. Cambridge, MA: Brookline Books, 1982. A thorough book that examines due process procedures in special education.

Cutler, Barbara Coyne. *Unraveling the Special Education Maze: An Action Guide for Parents*. Champaign, IL: Research Press, 1981. A guide for parents on how to deal with the special education system and be a good advocate for their child.

Des Jardins, Charlotte. *How To Get Services By Being Assertive.* Chicago: Coordinating Council For Handicapped Children, 1980. A handbook about obtaining services for handicapped children. Contains suggestions on advocating for your child.

Des Jardins, Charlotte. *How To Organize An Effective Parent/Advocacy Group and Move Bureaucracies.* Chicago: Coordinating Council for Handicapped Children, 1980. A handbook on organizing parent advocacy groups and working for change in educational services for handicapped children.

Fuge, D.L. and Green, K.O. *Estate Planning for Retarded Persons and Their Families.* Atlanta, GA: University of Mississippi Law Center, 1982. Covers issues about government programs, wills, trusts, life insurance, etc. Good for any type of disability where the person may not be able to provide for himself.

Moore, Ralph J., Jr. *Handbook on Estate Planning for Families of Developmentally Disabled Persons in Maryland, The District of Columbia, and Virginia.* Baltimore: Maryland State Planning Council On Developmental Disabilities, 1981. A guide to estate planning for parents of exceptional children. Although written for the laws of two states and the District of Columbia, the general legal principles are usually applicable.

Mopsik, Stanley I. and Judith A. Agard, eds. *An Education Handbook for Parents of Handicapped Children.* Cambridge, MA: Brookline Books, 1985. A detailed review of the special education process.

Russell, L.M. *Alternatives: A Family Guide to Legal and Financial Planning for the Disabled.* Evanston, Ill: First Publications, 1983. Presents how to plan for your child with mental disabilities. Covers everything from wills, trusts, government benefits, taxes and financial planning. Helps families plan early in understandable terms.

Shrybman, James A. *Due Process in Special Education.* Rockville, Maryland: Aspen Systems Corp., 1982. A detailed legal guide to the law and special education, including IEP, appeals, and due process hearings.

Stotland, Janet F., Esq. & Ellen Mancusco. *The Right to Special Education in Pennsylvania: A Guide for Parents.* Philadelphia: Education Law Center, Inc., 1984. Despite the title, a general booklet about the right to education of handicapped children.

Turnbull, H. & Turnbull, A.P. *Free Appropriate Public Education: Law and Implementation.* Denver: Love Publishing Co., 1982. Parents of disabled child (an attorney and special education teacher) discuss education opportunities for special needs kids. Specific information and a detailed presentation of rights are presented, as well as steps for parents to take to get an appropriate education.

United States Department of Education. *"To Assure the Free Appropriate Public Education of All Handicapped Children:" Seventh Annual Report to Congress on the Implementation of The Education of the Handicapped Act.* Office of Special Education and Rehabilitative Services, United States Department of Education, 1985. The annual report about Public Law 94–142, and about what is being done, or not being done, to carry out its purpose.

Chapter 9

Abrams, Bernard S. and Mike Hardin. *Fight for Life.* Columbus, OH: Silverwood Press (5510 Huntley Rd. Columbus, OH 43229), 1987. True story of man advocating for his daughter and getting a seizure medication from overseas.

Ballard, Joseph, Bruce Ramirez and Kathy Zantal-Wiener. *Public Law 94–142, Section 504, and Public Law 99–457 – Understanding What They Are and What They Are Not, 1987.* Available from Council for Exceptional Children, 1920 Association Drive, Reston, VA 22091-1589. A question and answer format that discusses all the recent changes in legislation that effect our children's educational rights.

Children's Defense Fund. *A Children's Defense Budget.* 122 C Street, NW, Washington, DC 20001, 1987. An in-depth examination of the federal programs and policies that affect children and families. Includes a section on ways to influence Congress' budgetmaking process and a guide to how the budget is made up. Also has trends in federal spending for child-serving programs. Good basic background for advocacy on the hill.

Children's Defense Fund. *Nonpartisan Voting Record of 1986.* 122 C St., NW, Washington, DC 20001, 1987. The voting record of members of the House and Senate on family and children's issues.

Children's Defense Fund. *It's Time to Stand Up for Your Children: A Parent's Guide to Child Advocacy.* 122 C St., NW, Washington, DC 20001, 1982. 48 page booklet, self-explanatory title.

Coelho, Tony. "Congressman Makes His Own Epilepsy a Campaign Issue to Break the Old Taboos." *People Magazine* 16, August 17, 1981. by Crawford-Mason. An interview with Congressman Coelho about his experience with epilepsy and his career.

Jordan, June B. and Bruce A. Ramirez. *1986 Special Education Yearbook.* Comprehensive resource that summarizes public policy, current issues, leaders in the field, statistical information etc. A thorough guide to everything you want to know about special education. Available from the Council for Exceptional Children, 1920 Association Drive, Reston, VA 22091-1589.

Guides, Newsletters, Periodicals, And Catalogs

Association for the Care of Children's Health (ACCH) *Books for Children and Teenagers About Hospitalization, Illness, and Disabling Conditions.* 1987 Edition. A greatly expanded update of the 1984 edition, this annotated bibliography describes more than 400 books and pamphlets for children and adolescents that deal directly or indirectly with some aspect of illness, hospitalization, or disabling conditions. Listed alphabetically by author's last name, each listing provides information on the publisher, identifies the book as fiction or nonfiction, suggests the approximate age group for which the book is intended, and provides a short content description. A topical index provides access to the listings by subject area.

Danmar Products, Inc. 2390 Winewood, Ann Arbor, Mich. 48103. Catalog with adaptive equipment, swimming aids, headgear, positioning aids, etc. Outstanding selection. Especially note the dolls with helmets for your child who must wear a helmet. Highly recommended.

Directory of Information Resources for the Handicapped: A Comprehensive Guide to Information Resources and Sources for the Handicapped. Written by the staff of Ready Reference Press, Santa Monica, CA, 1980. This directory lists the organization with its address and phone number and an in-depth description of the services provided. Very comprehensive. A list of directories is also included.

Durgin, Rod W., Lindsay, Norene, and Hamilton, Ellen. *The Guide to Recreation, Leisure and Travel for the Handicapped. Volume I: Recreation and Sports.* Toledo, OH: Resource Directories, 1985. Another everything you ever wanted to know resource. Recommended for the invaluable leads on toys and crafts that have been modified for special needs.

The Exceptional Parent. Boston: Psy-Ed Corporation & University of Boston School of Education. A useful and informative magazine for parents of special needs children. Recommended.

Growing Child. 22 North 2nd Street, PO 620, Lafayette, IN 47902. Newsletter sent each month beginning at birth up to age five. Each month describes developmental stages, educational play ideas, as well as specific behaviors to expect with age. Also included is a newsletter for parents called "Growing Parent." A must. Highly recommended.

Kapit, Wynn and Lawrence M. Elson. *The Anatomy Coloring Book.* New York, NY: Harper and Row, 1977. Clearly written text detailing human anatomy in coloring book format.

Katz, A.H. and K. Martin. *A Handbook of Services for the Handicapped.* Westport, CT: Greenwood Press, 1982. Comprehensive resource of the services available for physical care, housing, financial aid, employment, vocational rehabilitation, counseling, recreation and social activities, and special services for children.

National Information Center for Handicapped Children and Youth.P.O. Box 1492, Washington, DC 20013. Write and ask for the NICHCY Publication list. There are issue papers on many subjects ranging from Self-Advocacy, The Parent/Professional Partnership, to fact sheets on Learning Disabilities and Epilepsy. A great resource for educational materials if you want a break from reading books.

People First – A Reference Guide Regarding People with Disabilities. Contains suggestions for interacting with people with disabilities, useful glossary, list of common acronyms. North Carolina Council on Developmental Disabilities, Suite 615, 325 N. Salisbury St., Raleigh, NC 27611.

Slovak, Irene. *BOSC Directory. Facilities for Learning Disabled People.* Conger, NY. BOSC publishers, 1985. This resource guide is organized by states. It lists schools and independent living programs. The introduction and following articles are worth finding the directory to read. Extremely moving, educational, and inspirational.

Strobel, Susan. *Different? Understanding Epilepsy.* Greater Kansas City Epilepsy League. This workbook is full of puzzles, games, etc. about epilepsy. To order: Greater Kansas Epilepsy League, 4049 Pennsylvania, Suite 208, Kansas City, Missouri 64111.

What Happens After High School For Children With Disabilities?

Fielding, P.M. *A National Directory of Four Year Colleges, Two Year Colleges, and Post High School Training Programs for Young People with Learning Disabilities.* Tulsa, Okla: Partners in Publishing, 1984.

Liscio, M.A. *A Guide to Colleges for Learning Disabled Students.* Orlando, FL: Grune & Stratton, 1984.

Mangrum, C.T.,II and S.S. Strichart. *College and the Learning Disabled Student.* Orlando, FL: Grune & Stratton, 1984.

Ridenour, D.M. and J. Johnston. *A Guide to Post-Secondary Educational Opportunities for the Learning Disabled.* Oak Park, IL: Time Out to Enjoy, 1981.

Scholastic Aptitude Test, Educational Testing Service. *Information for Students with Special Needs.* Services for Handicapped Students, CN 6602, Princeton, NJ 08541.

Audio Cassettes For Chapter 5

Available from Nightengale-Conant Corp. in Chicago. Call 1–800–323–5552 for a catalogue and ordering information.

Brandon, Nathaniel. *The Psychology of High Self-Esteem.* Dr. Brandon has written about high self-esteem for 20 years. In this tape he explains how self-esteem problems develop and how the individual can learn to solve these problems. The special importance of being honest with oneself and acknowledging and accepting all aspects of oneself is highlighted in a unique way.

Dyer, Wayne. *What Do You Really Want for Your Children?* Dr. Dyer, a famous self-help psychologist, spoke with over four thousand parents in preparing to write his book *What Do You Really Want for Your Children?* This tape series covers topics treated by the book, including how to learn self-parenting, to have high self-esteem, to take risks, to have peaceful lives, and to be self-disciplined. The focus (as in all of Dr. Dyer's work) is on developing strongly inner-directed children who have a strong sense of confidence in their own judgement and abilities.

Mowaad, Bob. *You're Nature's Greatest Miracle* (kids 5–9); *You've Got What It Takes* (kids 10–13); *Unlocking Your Potential* (kids 14–17). These three tape series are absolutely superb. Mr. Mowaad is a very energetic, wise, and funny man who relates beautifully to children and teenagers, and these live recordings of his talks to young people are entertaining and inspiring. The goal of all these tapes is to inspire youngsters with a sense of their own uniqueness and potential. Dr. Mowaad teaches young people how to use their minds to pursue their desires and goals. The program for teenagers is the best I've ever heard and is strongly recommended for parents with children with special needs.

Tracy, Brian. *The Psychology of Achievement.* This is a superb set of tapes for anyone interested in developing more of their potential. Mr. Tracy's suggestions for using visualization and verbal affirmations to develop a positive self-concept are echoed by almost everyone in the field.

Waitley, Dennis. *2005: A Child's Odyssey.* This tape series covers low self-esteem, how parents' self-esteem affects children, how to build self-esteem and how to discipline with love.

Available from Marko Enterprises, 1831 Fort Union Blvd., Salt Lake City, Utah 84121

Smith, Randall. *10 Steps To Raising Self-Esteem.* This is a recording of a live presentation to a group of parents. Mr. Smith discusses the way in which learning about the "epidemic of low self-esteem" changed the way he related to his children and he has plenty of good ideas. Especially useful will be his thoughts regarding helping children feel like they are an important part of their family.

Available from General Cassette Corp. 602/269–3111.

Maltz, Maxwell. *Secrets To Children's Success Goals.* Using the structure of a fantasy detective game, Mr. Maltz (the author of *Psychocybernetics*) teaches children how to utilize their power of visualization to meet their goals. These tapes instruct children in using which is probably the most powerful untapped resource available to children and adults for improving their lives – their visual imagination.

Available from B.L. Winch and Associates, 45 Hitching Post Drive, Bldg. 2, Rolling Hills Estates, CA 90274, 800–662–9662.

Canfield, Jack. *Self-Esteem: The Key To Success.* Mr. Canfield is well-known for his book on developing self-esteem in the classroom. This tape series offers a rationale and practical exercises for developing self-acceptance and self-liking. The last half of the series presents relaxation and guided meditation exercises designed to help people live increasingly calm, focused, and successful lives. This series may be of particular interest to people who are interested in spiritual development as it related to self-esteem.

Available from Psychology Today Tapes 1–800–345–8112.

Brandon, Nathaniel. *Building Your Self-Esteem.* This is a tape of an interview in which Dr. Brandon discusses many of the ideas treated in *The Psychology of High Self-Esteem.*

Burns, David. *Feeling Good About Yourself.* This single audio tape is of an interview with Dr. Burns who discusses many of the ideas presented in his book, *Feeling Good.*

RESOURCE GUIDE

National Organizations

This resource guide contains the names, addresses, phone numbers, and a very brief description of the services provided by the following national organizations that can be of help to you and your child. If you are not certain about whether or not to join any of these organizations, call or write them and ask for their brochures, and a copy of their newsletter to help you decide.

ASSOCIATION FOR THE CARE OF CHILDREN'S HEALTH
3615 Wisconsin Ave. NW
Washington, DC 20016
202/244–1801
This organization is a leader in meeting the psychological and developmental needs of children and families in the health care setting through education, advocacy, and research programs. They have a bi-monthly newsletter and an excellent Parent Resource Guide which lists parents in each state. They also have a large selection of publications.

ASSOCIATION FOR RETARDED CITIZENS
2501 Avenue J
Arlington, TX 76011
871/640–0204
A grass roots national organization of advocates for retarded and special needs citizens. Publishes information about all types of developmental delays, advocates on behalf of retarded citizens and supports an extensive network of local associations. Each state ARC is listed in the local lists, however, you might find a county ARC nearer you. Look in your phone book. This organization offers diverse services and is a valuable contact.

ASSOCIATION FOR CHILDREN AND ADULTS WITH LEARNING DISABILITIES
4156 Library Road
Pittsburgh, PA 15234
412/341–1515
A grass roots national organization with over five hundred local offices meeting the needs of people with learning disabilities including information, advocacy, school program development, legislative action, and publications.

CHILDREN'S DEFENSE FUND
122 C St. NW
Washington, DC 20001
202/628-8787
An advocacy organization that focuses on the needs of children and families and is a strong, effective voice on Capitol Hill. Excellent publications.

COUNCIL FOR EXCEPTIONAL CHILDREN
1920 Association Drive
Reston, VA 22091-1589
703/620-3660
An organization made up of 954 local chapters directed toward the educational needs of exceptional children. Excellent publications, products, computer searches, etc.

THE EPILEPSY FOUNDATION OF AMERICA
4351 Garden City Drive
Landover, MD 20785
301/459-3700
800/EFA-1000
The foundation and its services have been thoroughly described in Chapter 10. However, the toll free number which can be reached from all area codes except 301, is a good first contact. The education, information, and referral provided is very comprehensive and remarkably up-to-date. Basic information about epilepsy can be obtained as well as more technical information which is backed up by the National Epilepsy Library and Resource Center. There are professionals on staff available to discuss various issues. You can also get referrals to other agencies and organizations, depending on your specific needs.

JOSEPH P. KENNEDY FOUNDATION
1350 New York Avenue, NW
Suite 500
Washington, DC 20005
202/393-1250
This foundation created and sponsors "Special Olympics." Of special interest is the "Let's Play to Grow" program which sponsors events for parents and infants that encourage early play activities. Write for *Discover,* the newsletter of "Let's Play to Grow."

KIDS ON THE BLOCK
9385 C Gerwig Lane
Columbia, MD 21046
301/290–9095
800/368–KIDS
This is a performing arts puppet show that gears its shows to school age children. The puppets have a variety of handicaps including epilepsy. Schools and PTA groups like the program very much. KIDS is organized in 49 of the 50 states.

MAINSTREAM
1200 15th St. NW
Washington, DC 20005
202/833–1136
This organization's motto is "Moving persons with disabilities into the workplace." Publishes a bimonthly newsletter about mainstreaming and has "Focus On" publications about various disabilities, including epilepsy.

THE NATIONAL EPILEPSY LIBRARY AND RESOURCE CENTER
4351 Garden City Drive
Landover, MD 20785
301/459–3700
This is the epilepsy library and resource center located at the national office of the Epilepsy Foundation. You can call or write for information, copies of articles, and virtually anything on any issue relating to epilepsy.

NATIONAL INFORMATION CENTER FOR HANDICAPPED CHILDREN AND YOUTH
7926 Jones Branch Drive
McLean, VA 22102
703/893–6061 800/999–5599
This organization provides free information to parents of handicapped children. It will answer specific questions, make referrals, provide information packets and fact sheets on a wide variety of disabilities.

SIBLING INFORMATION NETWORK
Department of Educational Psychology
Box U-64
The University of Connecticut
Storrs, CT 06268
203/486–4031
A clearinghouse of information on the disabled and their families with a concentration on siblings. Quarterly issues of a newsletter contain reviews, resource information, and discussions of family issues.

SIBLINGS FOR SIGNIFICANT CHANGE
823 United Nations Plaza
Room 808
New York, NY 10017
212/420–0776
An organization for siblings of the disabled. It provides information and referral services, access to legal aid, counseling programs, and community education.

Local Contacts

We want to thank the National Information Center for Handicapped Children and Youth for providing the information for the following state lists.

The agencies listed below are responsible for providing certain kinds of assistance to people with special needs and their families. One of the best resources for finding help for your child is your local school district. If your child is already in school and you think she needs special services, begin by discussing her needs with her teacher.

THE STATE DEPARTMENT OF EDUCATION can answer questions about how to get special education services in your state. Many states have special manuals explaining the steps to take. Check to see if one is available. State education officials need to know if your child is not receiving services or has problems because of inadequate services. This office usually has an ombudsman to assist you if you're having problems at the local level.

THE OFFICE OF VOCATIONAL EDUCATION FOR HANDICAPPED STUDENTS can tell you how the funds allocated to each state from the federal government are being used for vocational education for special needs students. They can also tell you what new programs you can expect.

THE PROTECTION AND ADVOCACY OFFICES are set up for people of all ages who have developmental disabilities. Services do vary from state to state. However, they will tell you what education, health, residential, social, and legal services are available. They basically have been established to protect the rights of handicapped people.

DEVELOPMENTAL DISABILITIES AGENCY has been designed to provide funding for direct services for people with developmental disabilities. Most of the programs are administered by private, nonprofit agencies and may provide such services as diagnosis, evaluation, recreation, group homes, information, and referral, social services, advocacy and protection.

THE STATE VOCATIONAL REHABILITATION AGENCY provides medical, therapeutic, counseling, education, training and other services needed to prepare people for work. The state agency will provide you with the nearest office to you.

Remember, in your search for information and referral, if the person you talk with can't help you, ask to be referred to someone else. Keep writing and phoning until you have the help you need. Keep a notebook beside the phone and log in each call. Jot down the date, phone number, agency, and person you talked with and what you talked about. You will be surprised at how useful it is to use as a reference later on.

State By State Resource List

ALABAMA

Program for Exceptional Children and
  Youth
Department of Education
1020 Monticello Court
Montgomery, AL 36117
205/261–5099
1–800/392–8020
Contact: Anne Ramsey, Coordinator

Special Needs Programs
Division of Vocational Education
  Services
Department of Education
806 State Office Bldg.
Montgomery, AL 36130
205/261–5224
Contact: Tom Pierce, Coordinator

Developmental Disabilities Planning
  Council
Department of Mental Health and
  Mental Retardation
200 Interstate Park Dr.
Montgomery, AL 36193-5001
205/271–9278
Contact: Joan Hannah, Executive
  Director

Alabama Developmental Disabilities
  Advocacy Program
The University of Alabama
P.O. Drawer 2847
Tuscaloosa, AL 35487-2847
205/348–4928
1–800/826–1675
Contact: Suellen R. Galbraith,
  Program Director

Alabama Council on Epilepsy, Inc.
Birmingham, AL
205/933–1471

Epilepsy Chapter of Mobile and Gulf
Coast
Mobile, AL
205/432–0970

Alabama Association for Children
with Learning Disabilities
P.O. Box 11588
Montgomery, AL 36111
205/277–9151

Mental Health Association in Alabama
306 Whitman St.
Montgomery, AL 36104
205/834–3857
Contact: Edna Earle Eich, Executive
Director

Alabama Association for Retarded
Citizens
444 South Decatur
Montgomery, AL 36105
205/262–7688
Contact: Douglas Sanford, Executive
Director

Alabama Easter Seal Society
2125 E. South Blvd.
Montgomery, AL 36199
205/288–8382
Contact: Barry F. Cavan, Executive
Vice President

ALASKA

Exceptional Children & Youth
Department of Education
Pouch F
Juneau, AK 99811
907/465–2824
Contact: William S. Mulnix, State
Director

Career and Vocational Education
Pouch F
Juneau, AK 99811
907/465–2980
Contact: Dr. Carole Veir, Program
Manager, Special Needs

Developmental Disabilities Section
Department of Health and Social
Services
Pouch H-04
Juneau, AK 99811
907/465–3372
Contact: Robert P. Gregovich,
Ph.D., Program Administrator

P&A for the Developmentally
Disabled, Inc.
325 E. 3rd Ave., 2nd Fl.
Anchorage, AK 99501
907/274–3658
Contact: David Maltman, Director

Alaska Association for Children with
Learning Disabilities
P.O. Box 60732
Fairbanks, AK 99706
907/479–4790
Contact: Roberta Wallace, President

Alaska Association for Retarded
Citizens
3605 Arctic Blvd., Suite 323
Anchorage, AK 99506
907/277–6677
907/338–5316
Contact: Robert M. Neely, President

Epilepsy Society
P.O. Box 9-2933
Anchorage, AK 99509
Contact: Rita Thompson

Special Education Parent Team for
Equal Rights
218 Front Street
Juneau, AK 99801
907/586–6806
Contact: Linda Griffith

ARIZONA

Division of Special Education
Department of Education
1535 W. Jefferson
Phoenix, AZ 85007
602/255–3183
Contact: Diane Petersen, Deputy
Associate Superintendent

Arizona Child Find Project
Department of Education
1535 W. Jefferson
Phoenix, AZ 85007
602/255–3183
Contact: Rita Kenison, Director

Education Program Support
Department of Education
Division of Vocational Education
1535 W. Jefferson
Phoenix, AZ 85007
602/255–5660

Contact: Jerry Bowman, Director
Governor's Council on
Developmental Disabilities
P.O. Box 6123 074Z
Phoenix, AZ 85005
602/255–4049
Contact: Jon C. Hinz, Executive
Director

Arizona Center for Law in the Public
Interest
112 N. Central Ave.
Suite 400
Phoenix, AZ 85004
602/252–4904
Contact: Amy J. Gittler, Executive
Director

Epilepsy Society of Central Arizona
Phoenix, AZ
602/265–1733

Association for Children with
Learning Disabilities
P.O. Box 15525
Phoenix, AZ 85060
602/840–3192

Mental Health Association of Arizona
1515 E. Osborn Rd., #18
Phoenix, AZ 85014
602/274–0527
Contact: John Simer, Director

Easter Seal Society of Arizona
903 No. 2nd St.
Phoenix, AZ 85004
602/252–6061
Contact: Gene Brantner, Executive
Director

Pilot Parents, Inc.
Central Palm Plaza - Suite 100
2005 N. Central Avenue
Phoenix, AZ 85004
602/271–4012

ARKANSAS

Special Education Division
Department of Education
Special Education Bldg., Room 105
Little Rock, AR 72201
501/371-2161
Contact: Diane Sydoriak, Director

Department of Vocational Education
Executive Bldg., Suite 220
2020 West 3rd St.
Little Rock, AR 72205
501/371-2374
Contact: Mary Williams, Special
Needs Programs Supervisor

Governor's Developmental
Disabilities Planning Council
4815 W. Markham St.
Little Rock, AR 72201
501/661-2589
Contact: Cindy Hartsfield,
Coordinator

Advocacy Services, Inc.
Medical Arts Bldg., Suite 504
12th & Marshall Streets
Little Rock, AR 72202
501/371-2171
1-800/482-1174
Contact: Nan Ellen East, Executive
Director

Arkansas Epilepsy Society, Inc.
Little Rock, AR
501/666-1355

Association for Children with
Learning Disabilities
P.O. Box 7316
Little Rock, AR 72217
501/666-8777
Contact: Maybian C. Sloan,
Executive Director

Mental Health Association
624 Malvern Ave.
Hot Springs, AR 71901
501/321-2129
Contact: Erika Hanzlik, Executive
Director

ARC/Arkansas
6115 West Markham Room 107
Little Rock, AR 72205
501/661-9992
Contact: Kathleen Wallace,
Executive Director

Arkansas Easter Seal Society
2801 Lee Avenue
P.O. Box 5148
Little Rock, AR 72205
Contact: James Butler, Executive
Director

Arkansas Special Education Resource
Center
P.O. Drawer 3623
Little Rock, AR 72203
501/376-0377
1-800/482-8437
Contact: Kathy Balkman, Executive
Director

CALIFORNIA

Special Education Division
Department of Education
P.O. Box 944272
Sacramento, CA 94244-2720
916/323-4768
Contact: Dr. Shirley Thornton,
Director

Department of Rehabilitation
830 K Street Mall
Sacramento, CA 95814
916/445–3971
Contact: P. Cecie Fontanoza,
    Director

California State Council on
    Developmental Disabilities
1507 21st Street, Suite 320
Sacramento, CA 95814
916/322–8481
Contact: James Shorter, Executive
    Director

Protection and Advocacy, Inc.
2131 Capitol Avenue, Suite 100
Sacramento, CA 95816
916/447–3324
800/952–5746
Contact: Albert Zonca, Executive
    Director

Epilepsy Society of San Diego County
San Diego, CA
619/296–0161

Epilepsy Society of Central California
Fresno, CA
209/485–6242

Epilepsy Society of San Francisco
San Francisco, CA
415/474–9075

Contra Costa-Alameda Epilepsy
    League
Oakland, CA
415/893–6272

Los Angeles County Epilepsy Society
Los Angeles, CA
213/382–7337

Epilepsy Society of San Bernardino
San Bernardino, CA
714/884–3494

Riverside-Imperial Counties Epilepsy
    Society
Riverside, CA
714/686–9183

Mental Health Association in
    California
P.O. Box 162695
Sacramento, CA 95816
916/455–5232
Contact: Hank Besayne, Executive
    Director

California Association for Retarded
    Citizens
1414 "K" Street, 3rd Floor
Sacramento, CA 95814
916/441–3322
Contact: Theodore E. Johnson,
    Executive Director

Easter Seal Society of California
742 Market, Suite 202
San Francisco, CA 94102
415/391–2006
Contact: William Barrett, Executive
    Director

CONNECTICUT

Bureau of Special Education & Pupil
    Personnel Services
Department of Education
P.O. Box 2219
Hartford, CT 06145
203/566–3561
Contact: Tom B. Gillung, Chief

Vocational Programs for the
Handicapped & Disadvantaged
Department of Education
25 Industrial Park Rd.
Middletown, CT 06457
203/638–4069
Contact: David S. Gifford, Director

Office of P&A for Handicapped &
Developmentally Disabled Persons
90 Washington Street
East Hartford, CT 06106
203/566–7616
203/566–2102
TTY/1–800/842–7303
Contact: Eliot J. Dober, Executive
Director

Epilepsy Foundation of Greater
Hartford
East Hartford, CT
203/282–1638

Association for Children with
Learning Disabilities of
Connecticut
139 N. Main St.
W. Hartford, CT 06107
203/236–3953

Mental Health Association in
Connecticut
705 A New Britain Ave
Hartford, CT 06106
Contact: Beverly Walton, Executive
Director

Connecticut Association for Retarded
Citizens
45 South Main Street
West Hartford, CT 06103
203/233–3629
203/378–5726
Contact: Margaret Dignoti,
Executive Director

Easter Seal Society of Connecticut,
Inc.
P.O. Box 100, Jones Street
Hebron, CT 06248-0100
203/228–9438
Contact: John R. Quinn, Executive
Director

DISTRICT OF COLUMBIA

Division of Special Education and
Pupil Personnel Services
DC Public Schools
10th & H Sts. NW
Washington, DC 20001
202/724–4018
Contact: Doris A. Woodson, State
Director

Webster Administrative Unit
10th & H St., NW
Washington, DC 20001
202/724–2142
Contact: Robbie Walker King,
Preschool/Child Find Coordinator

Rehabilitation Services
Administration
Department of Human Services
605 G St. NW
Washington, DC 20001
202/727–3227
Contact: Katherine Williams,
Administrator

Information Center for Handicapped
Individuals
605 G St., NW
Washington, DC 20001
202/347–4986
Contact: Yetta W. Galiber, Executive
Director

Epilepsy Foundation for the National
Capital Area
Washington, DC
202/638–5229

DC Association for Children with
Learning Disabilities
P.O. Box 6350
Washington, DC 20015
202/244–5177

DC Mental Health Association
1628 16th St. NW
Washington, DC 20009
202/265–6363
Contact: Anita Shelton, Executive
Director

Association for Retarded Citizens
900 Varnum Pl. NE
Washington, DC 20017
202/636–2950
Contact: Vincent C. Gray, Executive
Director

Easter Seal Society for Crippled
Children
2800 13th St. NW
Washington, DC 20009
202/232–2342
Contact: Nancy Marconi, Executive
Director

Parents Reaching Out Service
DC General Hospital
Department of Pediatrics
4th Fl. West Wing
1900 Massachusetts Ave. SE
Washington, DC 20003
202/727–3866
Contact: Marsha Parker, Program
Director

DELAWARE

Exceptional Children/Special
Programs Division
Department of Public Instruction
P.O. Box 1402
Dover, DE 19903
302/736–5471
Contact: Carl M. Haltom, Director

Vocational Education/Exceptional
Children Program
Department of Public Instruction
P.O. Box 1402
Dover, DE 19903
302/736–4681
Contact: Adam W. Fisher, Supervisor

Developmental Disabilities
Protection and Advocacy System
913 Washington St.
Wilmington, DE 19801
302/575–0660
800/292–7980
Contact: Mary McDonough, Acting
Director

Delaware Epilepsy Association
Wilmington, DE
302/658–9847

Association for Children with
Learning Disabilities
613 W. 37th St.
Wilmington, DE 19802
302/762-6262
Contact: JoAnne Allen, President

Mental Health Association of
Delaware
1813 North Franklin St.
Wilmington, DE 19802
302/656-8308
Contact: Gary Wirt, Executive
Director

Delaware Association for Retarded
Citizens
P.O. Box 1896
Wilmington, DE 19899
302/764-3662
Contact: William T. Wiest, Executive
Director

Easter Seal Society of Del-Mar
2705 Baynard Blvd.
Wilmington, DE 19802
302/658-6417
Contact: Sandra Kother, Executive
Director

Parent Information Center of
Delaware
Newark Medical Bldg. Suite 5
327 E. Main St.
Newark, DE 19711
302/366-0152
Contact: Patricia Herbert Frunzi,
Director

FLORIDA

Bureau of Education for Exceptional
Students
Department of Education
Knott Building
Tallahassee, FL 32301
904/488-1570
Contact: Dr. Wendy Cullar, Bureau
Chief

Handicapped & Workstudy Program
Division of Vocational Education
Department of Education
Knott Building
Tallahassee, FL 32301
904/488-5965
Contact: William Wargo, Coordinator

Developmental Disabilities Council
1311 Winewood Blvd.
Building 1, Room 308
Tallahassee, FL 32301
904/488-4180
Contact: Joseph Kreiger,
Administrator

Governor's Commission on Advocacy
for Persons with Disabilities
Clifton Bldg., Room 209
2661 Executive Center Circle, W.
Tallahassee, FL 32301
904/488-9070
1-800/342-0823
Contact: Jonathan P. Rossman,
Director

Epilepsy Foundation of Florida
Orlando, FL
305/876-4848

Gulf Coast Epilepsy Foundation, Inc.
Tampa, FL
813/962-3613

Epilepsy Foundation of Southwest
   Florida
Sarasota, FL
813/953–5988

Epilepsy Society of NW Florida
Pensacola, FL
904/433–1395

Suncoast Epilepsy Assoc., Inc.
St. Petersburg, FL
813/576–9107

Epilepsy Assoc. of Central Florida
Orlando, FL
305/422–1416

Epilepsy Assoc. of Broward County
Ft. Lauderdale, FL
305/581–2924

St. John's River Epilepsy Foundation
Jacksonville, FL
904/731–3752

Epilepsy Assoc. of the Palm Beaches
West Palm Beach, FL
305/478–6515

Epilepsy Foundation of South Florida
Miami, FL
305/324–4949

Florida Association for Children with
   Learning Disabilities
3115 W. Grace Street
Punta Gorda, FL 33950
813/637–8957
Contact: Diane Harrington,
   Executive Secretary

Mental Health Association of Florida
345 S. Magnolia Drive
Suite A-13
Tallahassee, FL 32301
904/877–4707
Contact: Peter Butzin, Executive
   Director

Florida Association for Retarded
   Citizens
106 S. Bronough St.
Tallahassee, FL 32301
904/681–1931
Contact: Kingsley Ross, Executive
   Director

Florida Easter Seal Society
1010 Executive Center Dr., Suite 101
Orlando, FL 32803
305/896–7881
Contact: Robert Griggs, Executive
   Director

Parent Education Network/FL, Inc.
2215 East Henry Avenue
Tampa, FL 33610
813/238–6100
Contact: Nadine Johnson, Director

Parent to Parent of Florida
c/o UCP of Panama City
621 Kraft Avenue
Panama City, FL 32401
904/769–1593

GEORGIA

Program for Exceptional Children
State Department of Education
1970 Twin Towers East
205 Butler St.
Atlanta, GA 30334
404/656–2425
Contact: Joan Jordan, State Director

Division of Secondary Vocational Instruction
1770 Twin Towers East
Atlanta, GA 30334
404/656–2516
Contact: Milton G. Adams, Coordinator of Special Needs Programs

Georgia Council on Developmental Disabilities
878 Peachtree St. NE, Rm. 620
Atlanta, GA 30309
404/894–5790
Contact: Zebe Schmitt, Executive Director

Georgia Advocacy Office, Inc.
1447 Peachtree St. NE
Suite 811
Atlanta, GA 30309
404/885–1447
1–800/282–4538
Contact: Pat Powell, Executive Director

Georgia Chapter, EFA
Atlanta, GA
404/527–7155

Georgia Association for Children & Adults with Learning Disabilities
P.O. Box 29492
Atlanta, GA 30329
404/633–1236
Contact: Marilyn Principle, Executive Secretary

Mental Health Association of Georgia
1244 Clairmont Ave.
Suite 204
Decatur, GA 30030
404/634–2850
Contact: Holly Hayes, Executive Director

Georgia Association of Retarded Citizens
1851 Ram Runway, Suite 104
College Park, GA 30337
404/761–3150
Contact: Mildred Hill, Executive Director

Georgia Easter Seal Society
1900 Emery St. NW Suite 106
Atlanta, GA 30318
404/351–6551
Contact: Timothy Murl, Executive Director

Parent to Parent of Georgia
1644 Tullie Cir.
Suite 123
Atlanta, GA 30309
404/636–1449
Contact: Kathy Reynolds, Director

Parents Educating Parents
1851 Ram Runway, Suite 102
College Park, GA 30337
404/761–2745
Contact: Mildred Hill, Director

HAWAII

Special Education Section
Department of Education
3430 Leahi Ave.
Honolulu, HI 96815
808/737-3720
Contact: Miles S. Kawatachi, State
Director

Occupational Development &
Compensatory Education Section
Office of Instructional Services
Department of Education
941 Hind Iuka Dr.
Honolulu, HI 96821
808/373-2984
Contact: Thomas Hata Keyama,
Director

Community Services for the
Developmentally Disabled
Family Health Services Division
Department of Health
741 E. Sunset Ave., Rm. 209
Honolulu, HI 96816
808/732-0935
Contact: Ethel Yamene, Chief

Protection and Advocacy Agency
1580 Makaloa St. Suite 860
Honolulu, HI 96814
808/949-2922
EPO 7777 toll free
Contact: Patty Henderson, Executive
Director

Hawaii Epilepsy Society
Honolulu, HI
808/523-7705

Hawaii Association for Children with
Learning Disabilities
200 N. Vineyard Blvd., Suite 402
Honolulu, HI 96817
Contact: Ivalee Sinclair, Executive
Director

Mental Health Association in Hawaii
200 N. Vineyard Blvd. Suite 507
Honolulu, HI 96817
808/521-1846
Contact: Nancy Vitale, Executive
Director

Hawaii Association for Retarded
Citizens
245 North Kukui St.
Honolulu, HI 96817
808/536-2274
Contact: Ahmad Saidin, Executive
Director

Easter Seal Society of Hawaii
710 Green St.
Honolulu, HI 96813
808/536-1015
Contact: Bill Hindman, Executive
Director

IDAHO

Special Education Division
Len B. Jordan Bldg.
650 W. State St.
Boise, ID 83720
208/334-3940
Contact: Martha Noffsinger, State
Director

Board for Vocational Education
650 W. State St.
Boise, ID 83720
208/334–3271
Contact: Mr. Roger Sathre,
  Supervisor of Special Needs

Bureau of Developmental Disabilities
Division of Community Rehabilitation
Department of Health & Welfare
450 W. State, 10th Fl.
Boise, ID 83720
208/334–4181
Contact: Paul Swatsenbarg, Ph.D.,
  Chief

Idaho's Coalition of Advocates for the
  Disabled, Inc.
W. Washington St.
Boise, ID 83702
208/336–5353
1–800/632–5125
Contact: Brent Marchbanks, Director

Idaho Epilepsy League
Boise, ID
208/344–4340

Mental Health Association in Idaho
715 S. Capitol Blvd., #401
Boise, ID 83702-7123
208/343–4866

ILLINOIS

Department of Specialized
  Educational Services
100 North First Street
Springfield, IL 62777
217/782–6601
Contact: Jonah Deppe, Special
  Education Specialist

Department of Adult, Vocational and
  Technical Education
Illinois State Board of Education
100 North First Street
Springfield, IL 62777
217/782–4870
Contact: James Galloway, Assistant
  State Superintendent

Governor's Planning Council on
  Developmental Disabilities
840 S. Spring Street
Springfield, IL 62706
217/782–9696
Contact: Carl Suter, Executive
  Director

Protection and Advocacy, Inc.
175 W. Jackson Blvd., Suite A-2103
Chicago, IL 60604
312/341–0022
Contact: Zena Naiditch, Executive
  Director

Epilepsy Services of Chicago
Chicago, IL
312/332–4107

Epilepsy Services for NE Illinois
Highland Park, IL
312/433–8960

Epilepsy Association of SW Illinois
Belleville, IL
618/398–0680

Lincoln Land Epilepsy Association
Springfield, IL
217/789–2258

Blackhawk Chapter Epilepsy
  Association
Moline, IL
309/762–3668

Epilepsy Association of DeKalb
County
DeKalb, IL
815/756–8554

Rock River Valley Epilepsy
Association
Rockford, IL
815/964–2689

Illinois Association For Children with
Learning Disabilities
20 E. Jackson St. Room 900
Chicago, IL 60604
312/663–9535
Contact: Mary Cotter

Mental Health Association in Illinois
217 E. Monroe St.
Springfield, IL 62701
Contact: Ann Nerod, President

Association for Retarded
Citizens-Illinois
600 S. Federal Street, Suite 123
Chicago, IL 60605
312/922–6932
Contact: Donald Moss, Executive
Director

Coordinating Council for
Handicapped Children
220 S. State Street, Rm. 412
Chicago, IL 60604
312/939–3513
Contact: Charlotte Des Jardins,
Director

INDIANA

Department of Education
Division of Special Education
Room 229 State House
Indianapolis, IN 46204
317/927–0216
Contact: Paul Ash, Acting Director

Governor's Planning Council on
Developmental Disabilities
Department of Mental Health
117 East Washington St.
Indianapolis, IN 46204
317/232–7820
Contact: Suellen Jackson-Boner,
Executive Director

Indiana Advocacy Services
850 N. Meridian St., Suite 2-C
Indianapolis, IN 46204
317/232–1150
1–800/622–4845
Contact: Ramesh K. Joshi, Executive
Director

Epilepsy Education Group of E.
Central Indiana
Muncie, IN
317/284–5035

Mental Health Association of Indiana
1433 N. Meridan St. Suite 203
Indianapolis, IN 46202
317/638–3501
Contact: Marilyn Schultz, President

Association for Retarded Citizens of
Indiana
110 E. Washington St., 9th Fl.
Indianapolis, IN 46204
317/632–4387
Contact: John Dickerson, Executive
Director

Indiana Association for Children with
  Learning Disabilities
508 Glade Place
Valparaiso, IN 46383
Contact: Cheryle Gunderson,
  President

Indiana Easter Seal Society for
  Crippled Children & Adults
3816 East 96th Street
Indianapolis, IN 46240
317/844-7919
Contact: James Carter, Executive
  Director

Task Force on Education for the
  Handicapped
Parent Advocacy Group
812 E. Jefferson Blvd.
South Bend, IN 46617
219/234-7101
Contact: Richard Burden, Director

IOWA

Division of Special Education
Department of Public Instruction
Grimes State Office Building
Des Moines, IA 50319
515/281-3176
Contact: J. Frank Vance, State
  Director

Rehabilitation, Education and
  Services Branch
Department of Public Instruction
510 E. 12th Street
Des Moines, IA 50319
515/281-4156
Contact: Mr. Jerry L. Starkweather,
  Associate Superintendent and
  Director

Governor's Planning Council for
  Developmental Disabilities
Division of MH/MR/Developmental
  Disabilities
Department of Human Services
Hoover State Office Building
Des Moines, IA 50319
515/281-7632
Contact: Karon Perlowski,
  Coordinator

Iowa Protection and Advocacy
  Service, Inc.
3015 Merle Hay Road, Suite 6
Des Moines, IA 50310
515/278-2502
Contact: Mervin Roth, Director

Epilepsy Association of Area VII
Waterloo, IA
319/236-4585

Iowa Association for Children with
  Learning Disabilities
R.R. #1, P.O. Box 116
Garner, IA 50438
515/923-2229
Contact: Arlene Greiman

Iowa Association for Retarded
  Citizens
715 E. Locust
Des Moines, IA 50309-1915
515/283-2358
1-800/367-2927
Contact: Mary Etta Lane, Executive
  Director

Iowa Federation–Council for
  Exceptional Children
240 Pickardy Lane
Council Bluffs, IA 51501
712/322-8336
Contact: Wilda Briggs, Director

Iowa Pilot Parents
1602 Tenth Avenue North
Fort Dodge, IA 50501
515/576–5870
800/362–2183
Contact: Carla Lawson, Director

KANSAS

Division of Special Education
State Department of Education
120 E 10th Street
Topeka, KS 66612
913/296–7454
Contact: Lucille Paden, Education
    Program Specialist

Vocational Education
State Department of Education
120 E. 10th St.
Topeka, KS 66612
913/296–4921
Contact: Ms. Carolyn Olson,
    Program Specialist

Planning Council for Developmental
    Disabilities
State Office Bldg., 5th Fl.
Topeka, KS 66612
913/296–2608
Contact: John Kelly

Advocacy & Protective Service for
    the Developmental Disabilities,
    Inc.
513 Leavenworth St., Suite 2
Manhattan, KS 66502
913/776–1541
800/432–8276
Contact: Joan Strickler, Executive
    Director

Epilepsy Kansas, Inc.
Wichita, KS
316/269–2526

Kansas Association for Children with
    Learning Disabilities
1727 W. 21st.
Lawrence, KS 66044
913/537–3880
Contact: Norma Dyck, President

Mental Health Association in Kansas
1205 Harrison
Topeka, KS 66612
913/357–5119
Contact: Kay Mettner, Executive
    Director

Kansas Association for Retarded
    Citizens
11111 West 59th Terrace
Shawnee, KS 66203
913/268–8200
Contact: Brent Glazier, Executive
    Director

Goodwill Industries - Easter Seal
    Society of Kansas
3636 N. Oliver
Wichita, KS 67220
316/744–0483
Contact: Marie Abney, President

KENTUCKY

Office of Education for Exceptional
    Children
Capital Plaza Tower, 8th Floor
Frankfort, KY 40601
502/564–4970
Contact: Vivian Link, Association
    Superintendent

Office of Vocational Rehabilitation
Services
Department of Education
Capital Plaza Tower, 9th Fl.
Frankfort, KY 40601
502/564-4440
Contact: Donald Fightmaster,
Association Superintendent

Kentucky Developmental Disabilities
Planning Council
Department For Mental
Health/Mental Retardation
Services
State Department of Human
Resources
275 East Main St.
Frankfort, KY 40621
502/564-7842
Contact: Rich Eversman, Director

Office For Public Advocacy
P&A Division
151 Elkorn Ct.
Frankfort, KY 40601
502/564-2967
1-800/372-2988 Developmental
Disabilities
Contact: Gayla Peach, Director

Kentucky Association for Children
with Learning Disabilities
2233 Alta Avenue
Louisville, KY 40205
502/451-8011
Contact: Catherine N. Senn,
President

Kentucky Association for Mental
Health
310 W. Liberty St. Suite 106
Louisville, KY 40202
502/585-4161
Contact: Ashar Tullis, Executive
Director

Kentucky Association for Retarded
Citizens
833 E. Main Street, Box 275
Frankfort, KY 40601
502/875-5225

Kentucky Easter Seal Society for
Crippled Children & Adults
233 E. Broadway
Louisville, KY 40202
502/584-9781
Contact: Guion Miller, Executive
Director

LOUISIANA

Special Educational Services
State Department of Education
P.O. Box 94064
Baton Rouge, LA 70804-9064
504/342-3631
Contact: Elizabeth S. Borel, Assistant
Superintendent

Division of Vocational Rehabilitation
Office of Human Development
P.O. Box 94371 Baton Rouge, LA
70804-9371
504/342-2285
Contact: May Nelson, Director

Louisiana State Planning Council on
  Developmental Disabilities
721 Government St., Rm 202
Baton Rouge, LA 70802
504/342-6804
Contact: Anne Farber, Executive
  Director

Advocacy Center for the Elderly &
  Disabled
1001 Howard Ave., Suite 300A
New Orleans, LA 70113
504/5-2-2337
800/662-7705
Contact: Lois V. Simpson, Executive
  Director

Louisiana Epilepsy Association
Baton Rouge, LA
504/292-9800

Epilepsy Council of Southeast
  Louisiana
New Orleans, LA
504/523-3879

Epilepsy Council of Southwest
  Louisiana
Lake Charles, LA
318/433-8688

Louisiana Association for Children
  with Learning Disabilities
Rt. 4, Box 110
Arnaudville, LA 70512
318/754-5287
Contact: Karen LaGrange, President

Mental Health Association of
  Louisiana
6700 Plaza Drive, Suite 104
New Orleans, LA 70127
504/241-3462
Contact: Richard E. Hitt, Executive
  Director

Louisiana Association for Retarded
  Citizens
658 St. Louis St.
Baton Rouge, LA 70802
504/383-0742
Contact: Patsy Davies, Interim
  Executive Director

Easter Seal Society for Crippled
  Children and Adults
4631 W. Napoleon Ave.
Metairie, LA 70002
504/455-5533
Contact: Daniel Underwood,
  Executive Director

Southwest Louisiana Education &
  Referral Center, Inc.
P.O. Box 52763
Lafayette, LA 70505
504/232-HELP
Contact: Sally Kent

MAINE

Division of Special Education
State Department of Educational &
  Cultural Services
State House, Station #23
Augusta, ME 04333
207/289-3451
Contact: David Noble Stockford,
  State Director

Bureau of Rehabilitation Services
Department of Human Services
32 Winthrop St.
Augusta, ME 04330
207/289–2266
Contact: Diana Scully, Director

Developmental Disabilities Council
State Office Bldg., Rm. 411
Station No. 40
Augusta, ME 04330
207/289–3161
Contact: Peter Stowell, Executive
  Director

Advocates for the Developmentally
  Disabled
P.O. Box 5341
Augusta, ME 04330
207/289–5755
1–800/452–1948
Contact: Dean Crocker

Pine Tree Epilepsy Association
Portland, ME
207/772–7847

Maine Association For Children &
  Adults with Learning Disabilities
P.O. Box 395
Topsham, ME 04086
Contact: Linda Felle, President

Special-Needs Parent Information
  Network S.P.I.N.
P.O. Box 2067
Augusta, ME 04330
207/582–2504
1–800/325–0220
Contact: Stacia Carver & Virginia
  Steele, Co-Directors

MARYLAND

Division of Special Education
State Department of Education
200 W. Baltimore St.
Baltimore, MD 21201
301/333–2485
Contact: Martha J. Fields, State
  Director

Vocational Rehabilitation
Division of Vocational Rehabilitation
State Department of Education
200 W. Baltimore St.
Baltimore, MD 21201
301/333–2294
Contact: Richard A. Batterton,
  Assistant State Superintendent

Developmental Disabilities Council,
  Room 429
201 West Preston St.
Baltimore, MD 21201
301/225–5077
Contact: Catherine A. Raggio,
  Executive Director

Maryland Disability Law Center
2510 St. Paul Street
Baltimore, MD 21218
301/333–7600
Contact: David Chavkin

Epilepsy Association of Maryland
Baltimore, MD
301/435–1100

Epilepsy Association of the Eastern
  Shore
Salisbury,MD
601/543–0665

Maryland Association for Children
with Learning Disabilities
24 Old Elm Rd.
North East, MD 21901
301/398-6017
Contact: Dot Clark, President

Mental Health Association of
Maryland
323 East 25th Street
Baltimore, MD 21218
301/235-1178
Contact: Herbert S. Cromwell,
Executive Director

Maryland Association for Retarded
Citizens
5602 Baltimore National Pike
Baltimore, MD 21228
301/744-0255
Contact: William Baber, Executive
Director

Central Maryland Chapter
National Easter Seal Society
3700 Fourth Street
Baltimore, MD 21225
301/355-0100
Contact: Mark Whitley, Executive
Director

MASSACHUSETTS

STATE DEPARTMENT OF
EDUCATION
Division of Special Education
Quincy Center Plaza
1385 Hancock St.
Quincy, MA 02169
617/770-7468
Contact: Dr. Roger Brown, State
Director

Commissioner, Massachusetts
Rehabilitation Commission
Statler Office Building
20 Park Plaza
Boston, MA 02116
617/727-2172
Contact: Mr. Elmer C. Bartels

Massachusetts Developmental
Disabilities Council
One Ashburton Pl.
Boston, MA 02108
617/727-6374
Contact: Jody Shaw, Executive
Director

Developmental Disabilities Law
Center, Inc.
11 Beacon St., Suite 925
Boston, MA 02108
617/723-8455
Contact: William Crane, Executive
Director

Office for Children
150 Causeway
Boston, MA 02214
617/727-8900
Contact: Mary Kay Leonard,
Executive Director

Epilepsy Association of Greater
Boston
Boston, MA
617/542-2292

Massachusetts Association for
Children with Learning Disabilities
P.O. Box 28
West Newton, MA 02165
617/891-5009

Massachusetts Association for Mental
  Health
14 Beacon Street
Boston, MA 02108
617/742-7452

Massachusetts Association for
  Retarded Citizens
217 South Street
Waltham, MA 02154
617/891-6270
Contact: Mary Lou Maloney,
  Executive Director

Massachusetts Easter Seal Society
Denholm Bldg.
484 Main St.
Worcester, MA 01608
617/757-2756
1-800/922-8290 MA only
Contact: Richard La Pierre, President

Federation for Children with Special
  Needs
312 Stuart St., 2nd Fl.
Boston, MA 02116
617/482-2915
Contact: Martha Ziegler, Executive
  Director

MICHIGAN

Special Education Services
Department of Education
P.O. Box 30008
Lansing, MI 48909
517/373-1695
Contact: Dr. Edward Birch, Director

Special Populations, Programs, &
  Services
Voc-Tech Education Service
Department of Education
P.O. Box 30009
Lansing, MI 48909
517/373-3387
Contact: Mr. Robert S. Kennon,
  Supervisor

Department of Mental Health
Developmental Disabilities Council
Lewis Cass Bldg., 6th Fl.
Lansing, MI 48926
517/373-6443
Contact: Beth Ferguson, Executive
  Director

Michigan P&A Service
313 So. Washington Square, Suite
  050
Lansing, MI 48933
517/487-1755
1-800/292-5923 voice and TTY
Contact: Elizabeth W. Bauer,
  Executive Director

Michigan Association for Children
  and Adults with Learning
  Disabilities
20777 Randall, Suite 18
Farmington Hills, MI 48024
313/471-0790
Contact: Joyce E. Martin, Secretary

Mental Health Association in
  Michigan
15920 W. Twelve Mile Rd.
Southfield, MI 48076
313/557-6777
1-800/482-9534
Contact: Tom Sovine, Executive
  Director

Michigan Association for Retarded
Citizens
313 S. Washington Sq., Suite 310
Lansing, MI 48933
517/487–5426
1–800/292–7851
Contact: Harvey Zuckerberg,
Executive Director

Citizens Alliance to Uphold Special
Education
313 So. Washington Square, Suite
040
Lansing, MI 48933
517/485–4084 Voice/TDD
1–800-221-9105
Contact: Eileen M. Cassidy,
Executive Director

Easter Seal Society of Michigan
4065 Saladin Dr., SE
Grand Rapids, MI 49506
616/942–2081
Contact: Susan Quinn, Executive
Director

MINNESOTA

Special Education Section
State Department of Education
Capitol Square Bldg.
550 Cedar St.
St. Paul, MN 55101
612/296–4163
Contact: Norena A. Hale, Director

Division of Vocational Rehabilitation
Department of Economic Security
390 N. Roberts St, 5th Fl.
St. Paul, MN 55101
612/296–1822
Contact: William Niederloh,
Assistant Commissioner

Governor's Planning Council on
Development Disabilities
201 Capitol Square Bldg.
550 Cedar Street
St. Paul, MN 55101
612/296–4018
Contact: Colleen Wieck, Executive
Director

Legal Aid Society of Minneapolis
222 Grain Exchange Bldg.
323 Fourth Ave., South
Minneapolis, MN 55415
612/338–0968
1–800/292–4150
Contact: Jeremy Lane, Executive
Director

Epilepsy Foundation of Minnesota
St. Paul, MN
612/646–8675

Arrowhead Epilepsy League
Duluth, MN
218/722–4526

Minnesota Association for Children
with Learning Disabilities
1821 Univ. Ave., Rm. 494-N
St. Paul, MN 55104
612/646–6136
Contact: Gary Berg, Executive
Director

Mental Health Association of
Minnesota
328 E. Hennepin
2nd floor
Minneapolis, MN 55414
612/331–6840
1–800/862–1799
Contact: George Carr, Executive
Director

Minnesota Association for Retarded
  Citizens
3225 Lyndale Ave. South
Minneapolis, MN 55408-3699
612/827-5641
1-800/582-5256
Contact: James Rummel, Executive
  Director

Parent Advocate Coalition for
  Education Rights Center, Inc.
4826 Chicago Ave, South
Minneapolis, MN 55417-1055
612/827-2966
1-800/53--ACER
Contact: Marge Goldberg and Paula
  Goldberg, Co-Directors

MISSISSIPPI

Bureau of Special Services
Department of Education
P.O. Box 771
Jackson, MS 39205
601/359-3490
Contact: Dr. Walter H. Moore,
  Director

Department of Rehabilitation
  Services
932 North State St.
P.O. Box 1698
Jackson, MS 39215-1698
601/354-6825
Contact: Mr. Jerry Sawyer, Director

Developmental Disabilities
Department of Mental Health
1100 Robert E. Lee Bldg.
Jackson, MS 39201
691/359-1290
Contact: E.C. Bell, Director

Mississippi P&A System for the
  Developmentally Disabled
4793 B McWillie Drive
Jackson, MS 39206
601/981-8207
1-800/772-4057
Contact: Becky Floyd, Director

Epilepsy Foundation of Mississippi
Jackson, MS
601/362-2761

Mississippi Association for Children
  with Learning Disabilities
3825 Ridgewood Rd.
Jackson, MS 39211
601/982-6767
Contact: Dr. Rita Nordan, President

Mississippi Association for Retarded
  Citizens
813 West Pine St, Suite B
Hattiesburg, MS 39401
601/544-4039
Contact: Barbara Caperton,
  Executive Director

Mississippi Easter Seal Society
P.O. Box 4958
3226 N. State St.
Jackson, MS 39216
601/982-7051
Contact: Lee O. Dees, Executive
  Director

Client Assistant Program
Mississippi Easter Seal Society
P.O. Box 4958
3226 N. State St.
Jackson, MS 39216
601/982-7051
Contact: Wanda Kenney, Director

Association of Developmental
Organizations of Mississippi, Inc.
ADOM/6055 Highway 18 So.
Jackson, MS 39209
601/922–3210
Contact: Anne Presley, Executive
Director

MISSOURI

Division of Special Education
Department of Elementary and
Secondary Education
P.O. Box 480
Jefferson City, MO 65102
314/751–2965
314/751–3251
Contact: John Heskett, Coordinator

Vocational Special Needs and
Guidance Services
Department of Elementary and
Secondary Education
P.O. Box 480
Jefferson City, MO 65102
314/751–1394
Contact: Robert Larivee, Director

Department of Mental Health
P.O. Box 687
Jefferson City, MO 65102
314/751–4054
Contact: Kay Conklin, Coordinator

Missouri Protection and Advocacy
Services, Inc.
211 B Metro Drive
Jefferson City, MO 65101
314/893–3333
1–800/392–8667
Contact: Carol D. Larkin, Director

Greater Kansas City Epilepsy League
Kansas City, MO
816/276–8940

Epilepsy Federation of Greater St.
Louis
St. Louis, MO
314/645–6969

Missouri Association for Children
with Learning Disabilities
P.O. Box 3303
Glenstone Station
Springfield, MO 65804
Contact: Eleanor Scherff, Executive
Director

Mental Health Association in Missouri
Box 1667
Jefferson City, MO 65102
314/635–7139
Contact: Frances Bradley, Executive
Director

Missouri Easter Seal Society, Inc.
1000 Watson Rd., Suite 18
St. Louis, MO 63126
314/821–6001
Contact: Barbara Robinson,
Executive Director

MONTANA

Special Education Unit
Office of Public Instruction
State Capitol
Helena, MT 59620
406/444–4429
Contact: Gail Gray, State Director

Vocational Education Services
Office of Public Instruction
Helena, MT 59620
406/444–2413
Contact: Gene Christiansen,
   Assistant Superintendent

Developmentally Disabled Planning
   and Advisory Council
25 South Ewing
Helena, MT 59601
406/444–6825
Contact: Clyde Muirheid

Montana Advocacy Program Inc.
1219 East 8th Avenue
Helena, MT 59601
406/444–3889
Contact: Kristin Balula, Executive
   Director

Epilepsy Association of Southwest
   Montana
Butte, MT
406/723–4243

Montana Association for Children
   with Learning Disabilities
3024 Macona Lane
Billings, MT 59101
406/252–4845
Contact: Ellen Alweis, President

Mental Health Association of
   Montana
1030 N. Montana
Helena, MT 59601
406/442–4276
Contact: Liz Buck, Administrative
   Secretary

Montana Association for Retarded
   Children
2025 So. Billings Blvd.
Trailer Village, Lot #70
Billings, MT 59101
406/248–8249
Contact: Beverly Owens, President

Easter Seal Society - Goodwill
   Industries of Montana
4400 Central Avenue
Great Falls, MT 59401
406/761–3680
Contact: William Sirak, Executive
   Director

NEBRASKA

Special Education Branch
State Department of Education
P.O. Box 94987
Lincoln, NE 68509
402/471–2471
Contact: Gary Sherman, State
   Director

Vocational Special Needs Program
Division of Vocational Education
Department of Education
P.O. Box 94987
Lincoln, NE 68509-4987
402/471–4808
Contact: Steve A. Equall,
   Administrator

Developmental Disabilities Program
Department of Health
P.O. Box 95007
Lincoln, NE 68509
402/471–2330
Contact: Eric Evans, Director

Nebraska Advocacy Services for
  Developmentally Disabled
  Citizens, Inc.
522 Lincoln Center Building
215 Centennial Mall, Room 522
Lincoln, NE 68508
402/474–3183
Contact: Timothy Shaw, Executive
  Director

Epilepsy Association of Nebraska
Omaha, NE
402/342–0290

Nebraska ACLD
1421 Fairfield
Lincoln, NE 68521
402/435–2395
Contact: Linda Greder Vorisek,
  President

Mental Health Association of
  Nebraska
Lincoln Center Bldg #4B
215 Centennial Mall So.
Lincoln, NE 68508
402/476–8735

Nebraska Association for Retarded
  Citizens
502 Executive Building
521 South 14th Street
Lincoln, NE 68508
402/475–4407
Contact: David Powell, Executive
  Director

Easter Seal Society of Nebraska
3015 No. 90th St., Suite 6
Omaha, NE 68134
402/571–2162
Contact: Tish Simmons, Executive
  Director

NEVADA

Nevada Department of Education
Special Education Branch
400 W. King St.
Capitol Complex
Carson City, NV 89710
702/885–3140
Contact: Jane Early, State Director

Rehabilitation Division
Department of Human Resources
Kinkead Building, Fifth Floor
505 East King Street
Capitol Complex
Carson City, NV 89710
702/885–4440
Contact: Delbert E. Frost,
  Administrator

Developmentally Disabled Council
c/o Department of Rehabilitation
505 East King St., Rm. 502
Capitol Complex
Carson City, NV 89710
702/885–4440
Contact: Ken Vogel, Director

Developmentally Disabled
  Advocate's Office
2105 Capurro Way, Suite B
Sparks, NV 89431
702/789–0233
800/992–5715
Contact: Holli Elder, Project Director

Nevada Association for Children with
   Learning Disabilities
Box 188
Alamo, Nevada 89001
Contact: Kristin Thomas, President

Association for Retarded Citizens
680 S. Bailey St.
Fallon, NV 89406
702/423–4760
Contact: Frank Weinrauch,
   Executive Director

Easter Seal Society for Crippled
   Children and Adults of Nevada
1455 E. Tropicana Avenue, Suite 660
Las Vegas, NV 89119
702/739–7771
Contact: Nancy Kosik, Executive
   Director

NEW HAMPSHIRE

Special Education Bureau
Department of Education
101 Pleasant St.
Concord, NH 03301
603/271–3741
Contact: Robert T. Kennedy,
   Director of Special Education

Vocational Special Services
State Department of Education
Division of Voc-Tech Education
101 Pleasant St.
Concord, NH 03301
603/271–3186
Contact: John E. Bean, Jr. Consultant

State Developmental Disabilities
   Council
9 S. Spring St. Suite 204
Concord, NH 03301
603/271–3236
Contact: Susan Parker, Executive
   Director

Developmentally Disabled Advocacy
   Center, Inc.
6 White St.
P.O. Box 19
Concord, NH 03301
603/228–0432
1–800/852–3336
Contact: Donna Woodfin, Director

Central NH Community Mental
   Health Services
P.O. Box 2032
Concord, NH 03301
603/228–1551
Contact: Terje Reinertsen, Director

New Hampshire Association for
   Retarded Citizens
10 Ferry St.
Concord Center
Concord, NH 03301-5077
603/228–9092
Contact: Karen Cowan

Easter Seal Society-Goodwill
   Industries of New Hampshire
555 Auburn St.
Manchester, NH 03103
603/623–8863
Contact: Robert Cholette, Director

Parent Information Center
P.O. Box 1422
Concord, NH 03301
603/224–7005
Contact: Judith Raskin, Director

Upper Valley Support Group
Box 622
Hanover, NH 03755
603/448-6311
Contact: Bev Parry, Executive
Director

Special Families United
P.O. Box 5
New London, NH 03257
603/526-2716
Contact: Margaret Gay, President

NEW JERSEY

Division of Special Education
Department of Education
225 W. State St. CN 500
Trenton, NJ 08625
609/292-0147
Contact: Jeffery Osowski, Director

Division of Vocational Rehabilitation
Department of Labor and Industry
1005 Labor and Industry Bldg.
John Fitch Plaza, CN 398
Trenton, NJ 08625
609/292-5987
Contact: George R. Chizmadia,
Director

Statewide Computerized Referral
Information Program SCRIP
108-110 N. Broad St. CN 700
Trenton, NJ 08625
609/292-3745
1-800/792-8858 in NJ
Contact: Patricia Krupka,
Administrator

Department of Public Advocate
Division of Advocacy for the
Developmentally Disabled CN850
Trenton, NJ 08625
609/292-9742
Contact: Sarah W. Mitchell, Director

Epilepsy Foundation of New Jersey
Trenton, NJ
609/392-4900

New Jersey Association for Children
with Learning Disabilities
284 E. Main St.
Oceanport, NJ 07757
201/389-3337
Contact: Allen Goldberg, President

Mental Health Association in New
Jersey
60 South Fullerton Ave.
Montclair, NJ 07042
Contact: Carolyn Beauchamp,
Director

Association for Retarded Citizens
985 Livingston Ave.
North Brunswick, NJ 08902
201/246-2525
Contact: John Scagnelli, Executive
Director

Easter Seal Society of New Jersey
Box 155
32 Ford Ave.
Milltown, NJ 08850
201/247-8353
Contact: Clark Paradise, President

NEW MEXICO

Division of Special Education
State Department of Education
300 Don Gaspar Ave.
Santa Fe, NM 87501-2786
505/827–6541
Contact: Elie S. Gutierrez, State
    Director

Division of Vocational Rehabilitation
    Department of Education
604 W. San Mateo
Santa Fe, NM 87503
505/827–3511
Contact: Orlando J. Giron, Director

Developmentally Disabled Planning
    Council
Health Planning Development
    Division
Health and Environment Department
P.O. Box 968
Santa Fe, NM 87504-0968
Contact: James P. Crews, Acting
    Director

Protection and Advocacy System
201 San Pedro N.E.
Building 4, Suite 140
Albuquerque, NM 87110
505/888–0111
Contact: James Jackson, Executive
    Director

New Mexico Association for
    Retarded Citizens
8210 La Mirada, N.E.
Suite 500
Albuquerque, NM 87109
505/298–6796
Contact: Kermitt Stuve, Executive
    Director

Easter Seal Society of New Mexico
4805 Menaul NE
Albuquerque, NM 87110
505/888–3811
Contact: Tim Taschwer, Executive
    Director

NEW YORK

Office for Education of Children with
    Handicapping Conditions
State Department of Education
Education Bldg. Annex, Rm. 1073
Albany, NY 12234
518/474–5548
Contact: Lawrence Gloecker,
    Assistant Commissioner

Office of Vocational Rehabilitation
State Department of Education
1 Commerce Plaza
99 Washington Avenue, Rm. 1907
Albany, NY 12234
518/474–3981
Contact: Richard Switzer, Deputy
    Commissioner

Bureau of Occupational Education
Policy Development
State Education Department
One Commerce Plaza, Rm. 1624
Albany, NY 12234
518/473–7408
Contact: Barbara Shay, Chief

Developmental Disabilities Planning
    Council
1 Empire State Plaza, 10th Fl.
Albany, NY 12223
518/474–3655
Contact: Andrew D. Virgilio,
    Executive Director

Commission on Quality of Care for
the Mentally Disabled
99 Washington Ave, Suite 1002
Albany, New York 12210
518/473-7378
Contact: Clarence J. Sundram,
Commissioner

Epilepsy Society of New York City
New York, NY
212/967-2930

Epilepsy Foundation of Nassau
County
Garden City, NY
516/794-5500

New York State Epilepsy Association
New York, NY
212/684-3344

Epilepsy Society, Inc.
Suffern, NY
914/357-3490

Epilepsy Association of the Capital
District
Albany, NY
518/456-7501

New York Association for the
Learning Disabled
155 Washington Ave., 3rd Floor
Albany, NY 12210
518/436-4633
Contact: Pat Lilac, Executive
Director

Mental Health Association of NYS
196 Morton Ave.
Albany, NY 12002
518/449-5677
Contact: Leila Salmon, Director

New York State Association for
Retarded Children, Inc.
393 Delaware Ave.
Delmar, NY 12054
518/439-8311
Contact: Marc Brandt, Director

New York Easter Seal Society for
Crippled Children and Adults
845 Central Avenue
Albany, NY 12206
518/438-8785
Contact: David Timko, Executive
Director

NORTH CAROLINA

Division of Exceptional Children
Department of Public Instruction
114 E. Edenton St.
Raleigh, NC 27611
919/733-3921
Contact: Lowell Harris, State
Director

Division of Vocational Rehabilitation
Services
Department of Human Resources
620 North West Street
Post Office Box 26053
Raleigh, NC 27611
919/733-3364
Contact: Mr. Claude A. Myer,
Director

Council on Developmental
Disabilities
Department of Human Resources
1508 Western Boulevard
Raleigh, NC 27606
919/733-6566
Contact: James W. Keene, Director

Governor's Advocacy Council for
   Persons with Disabilities
1318 Dale St., Suite 100
Raleigh, NC 27605
919/733–9250
1–800/662–7030
Contact: Lockhart Follin-Mace,
   Director

Epilepsy Association of North
   Carolina
Raleigh, NC
919/834–2876

North Carolina Association for
   Children with Learning Disabilities
105 Juniper Place
Chapel Hill, NC 27514
919/967–6170 - office
919/493–4336 - home
Contact: Sharon Meginnis, President

Mental Health Association in North
   Carolina
5 West Hargett St., Suite 705
Raleigh, NC 27601
919/828–8145
Contact: Deva Wright, Executive
   Director

North Carolina Association for
   Retarded Citizens
2400-A Glenwood Avenue
Raleigh, NC 27608-1399
919/782–4632
Contact: Carey S. Fendley,
   Executive Director

Easter Seal Society of North Carolina
832 Wake Forest Rd.
Raleigh, NC 27604
919/834–1191
Contact: Edward Kershaw, Executive
   Director

Advocacy Center for Children's
   Education and Parent Training
P.O. Box 27952
Raleigh, NC 27611
919/821–2048
1–800/532–5358
Contact: Jennifer Seykora, Director

NORTH DAKOTA

Special Education Division
Department of Public Instruction
State Capitol
Bismarck, ND 58505
701/224–2277
800/932–8974
Contact: Dr. Gary Gronberg,
   Director

Board for Vocational Education
State Capitol
Bismarck, ND 58505
701/224–3178
Contact: Marcia Schutt, Supervisor of
   Special Needs

Developmental Disabilities Council
Department of Human Services
State Capitol
Bismarck, ND 58505
701/224–2970
Contact: Tom Wallner

P & A Project for the
   Developmentally Disabled
State Capitol Annex, 1st Floor
Bismarck, ND 58505
701/224–2972
800/472–2670
Contact: Barbara C. Braun, Director

North Dakota Association for
    Children with Learning Disabilities
2025 Ida Mae Ct.
Minot, ND 58701
701/839–6877
Contact: Doralyn Brown, President

North Dakota Mental Health
    Association
P.O. Box 160
Bismarck, ND 58502
701/225–3692
Contact: Myrt Armstrong, Executive
    Director

North Dakota Association for
    Retarded Citizens
418 E. Broadway Ave.
Bismarck, ND 58501
701/223–5349
Contact: Dan Ulmer, Executive
    Director

Easter Seal Society of North Dakota
Box 490
Bismarck, ND 58502
701/223–8730
Contact: Patricia Conrad, Executive
    Director

OHIO

Division of Special Education
State Department of Education
933 High St.
Worthington, OH 43085
614/466–2650
Contact: Frank E. New, Director

Ohio Rehabilitation Services
    Commission
4656 Heaton Rd.
Columbus, OH 43229
614/438–1210 voice/TTY
1–800/282–4536
Contact: Robert Rabe, Administrator

Office of Developmentally Disabled
    Council
Department of MR/Developmentally
    Disabled
Atlas Bldg.
8 East Long St.
Columbus, OH 43215
614/466–5205
Contact: Ken Campbell, Executive
    Director

Ohio Legal Rights Service
8 East Long St. 8th Fl.
Columbus, OH 43215
614/466–7264
1–800/282–9781
Contact: Carolyn Knight, Executive
    Director

Epilepsy Association of Central Ohio
Columbus, OH
614/228–4401

Epilepsy Center of Northwestern
    Ohio
Toledo, OH
419/241–5401

Epilepsy Foundation of Northeast
    Ohio
Dayton, OH
513/228–8401

Epilepsy Foundation of Northeast
Ohio
Cleveland, OH
216/579-1330

Ohio ACLD State Office
2800 Euclid Ave. Suite 308
Cleveland, OH 44115
216/861-6665
Contact: Mary Giallambardo,
President

Mental Health Association of Ohio
50 West Broad St., Suite 2440
Columbus, OH 43215
614/221-5383
Contact: Donald L. Farrow,
Executive Director

Ohio Association for Retarded
Citizens
360 S. 3rd St. Suite 101
Columbus, OH 43215
614/228-4412
Contact: Carolyn Sidwell, Executive
Director

Ohio Easter Seal Society, Inc.
2204 S. Hamilton Rd.
P.O. Box 32462
Columbus, OH 43232
614/868-9126
Contact: Prentis Wilson, Executive
Director

Citizens Advocacy Coalition
215 W. Rayon Ave.
Youngstown, OH 44583
Contact: Kathy Traynor, Chairperson

OKLAHOMA

Sec. for Exceptional Children
State Department of Education
2500 N. Lincoln, Suite 263
Oklahoma City, OK 73105
405/521-3351
Contact: Jimmie L.V. Prickett, State
Director

Division of Rehabilitation Services
Department of Human Services
P.O. Box 25352
Oklahoma City, OK 73125
405/424-4311 ext. 2840
Contact: A. C. Adams, Director

Developmental Disabilities Services
Department of Human Resources
P.O.Box 25352
Oklahoma City, OK 73125
405/521-3571
Contact: Jean Cooper, Assistant
Director

Protection and Advocacy Agency for
the Developmentally Disabled
9726 East 42nd St.
Osage Building, Room 133
Tulsa, OK 74146
918/664-5883
Contact: Bob M. Van Osdol, Director

Epilepsy Foundation of the Sooner
State
Oklahoma City, OK
405/521-1018

Oklahoma Association for Children
with Learning Disabilities
3701 NW, 62nd St.
Oklahoma City, OK 73112
405/943-9434
Contact: Jeanne Asher

Mental Health Association of
  Oklahoma
5104 N. Francis, Suite B
Oklahoma City, OK 73118
405/524-6363
Contact: Elizabeth Holmes,
  Executive Director

OASIS Handicapped Children's
  Information Hotline
3 Nicholson Tower, Rm. 360,OCMH
940 Northeast 13th St.
Oklahoma City, OK 73104
Contact: Pat Burns, Project Director

Easter Seal Society, Inc.
2100 NW 63rd St.
Oklahoma City, OK 73116
405/848-7603
Contact: Wallace Bonifield,
  Executive Director

PRO Oklahoma Parents Reaching
  Out in Oklahoma
2701 N. Portland
Oklahoma City, OK 73107
405/948-1618
Contact: Connie Motsinger, Director

OREGON

Special Education & Student
  Services Division
Department of Education
700 Pringle Parkway S.E.
Salem, OR 97310-0290
503/378-2677
Contact: Patricia Ellis, Associate
  Superintendent

Vocational Rehabilitation Division
Department of Human Resources
2045 Silverton Road, N.E.
Salem, OR 97310
503/378-3830
Contact: Joil A. Southwell,
  Administrator

Oregon Developmentally Disabled
  Planning Council
2575 Bittern St., N.E.
Salem, OR 97310-0520
503/378-2429
Contact: Russ Gurley

Oregon Advocacy Center
625 Board of Trade Bldg.
310 Southwest Fourth Ave.
Portland, OR 97204
503/243-2081
1-800/452-1694
Contact: Elam Lantz, Jr., Executive
  Director

Epilepsy Association of Oregon
Portland, OR
503/228-7651

Oregon Association for Children with
  Learning Disabilities
Portland State University
P.O. Box 751
Portland, OR 97207
503/229-4439
Contact: Evelyn Murphy, Executive
  Director

Mental Health Association in Oregon
718 W. Burnside St., Room 301
Portland, OR 97209
503/228-6571
1-800/452-5011
Contact: Shary White, Administrative
  Assistant

Oregon Association for Retarded
 Citizens
1745 State St., N.E.
Salem, OR 97301
503/581-2726
1-800/452-0313
Contact: Janna Starr, Executive
 Director

Easter Seal Society of Oregon
5757 SW Macadam
Portland, OR 97201
503/228-5108
Contact: Bill Hamilton, President

PENNSYLVANIA

Bureau of Special Education
333 Market St.
Harrisburg, PA 17126-0333
717/783-6913
Contact: Gary Makuch, State
 Director

Office of Vocational Rehabilitation
Department of Labor & Industry
Labor & Industry Building, Rm. 1300
7th and Forster Streets
Harrisburg, PA 17120
717/787-5244
Contact: George C. Lowe, Jr.,
 Executive Director

Developmentally Disabled Planning
 Council
569 Forum Bldg.
Harrisburg, PA 17120
717/787-6057
Contact: David B. Schwartz,
 Executive Director

Pennsylvania Protection and
 Advocacy, Inc.
3540 N. Progress Ave.
Harrisburg, PA 17110
717/657-3320
800/692-7443
Contact: Elmer Cerano, Executive
 Director

Epilepsy Foundation of Philadelphia
Philadelphia, PA
215/863-9581

Epilepsy Association of Lehigh Valley
Wind Gap, PA
215/863-9581

Epilepsy Foundation of Western
 Pennsylvania
Pittsburgh, PA
412/261-5880

Association for Children with
 Learning Disabilities
Toomey Bldg., Suites 2 & 3
P.O. Box 208
Uwchland, PA 19480
215/458-8193
800/692-6200
Contact: Mary Rita Hanley,
 Executive Director

Mental Health Association of
 Pennsylvania
900 Market Street
Harrisburg, PA 17101
715/255-2888

Pennsylvania Association for
Retarded Citizens
123 Forster St.
Harrisburg, PA 17102
717/234-2621
Contact: William A. West, Executive
Director

The Pennsylvania Easter Seal Society
P.O. Box 497
1500 Fulling Mill Rd.
Middletown, PA 17057-0497
717/939-7801
Contact: William E. Graffius, Director

Connect Information Service
Technical Assistance Group for Right
to Education
150 S. Progress Avenue
Harrisburg, PA 17109
800/692-7288

PUERTO RICO

Special Education Program
Department of Education
P.O. Box 759
Hato Rey, PR 00919
809/764-8059
Contact: Ms. Lucila Torres Martinez

Developmental Disabilities Council
P.O. Box 9543
Santurce, PR 00908
809/722-0590 or 0595
Contact: Mrs. Maria Luisa Mendia,
Acting Director

Protection and Advocacy
Department of Consumer Affairs
Minillas Governmental Center
North Building
P.O. Box 41059
Santurce, PR 00904
809/727-8880
Contact: Ms. Marianela Rosario,
Acting Director

Epilepsy Society of Puerto Rico
Bayamon, PR
809/782-6262

Puerto Rico Association for Children
with Learning Disabilities
G.P.O. Box 3521
San Juan, PR 00936
809/728-3635
Contact: Marie Lipuscek, President

Puerto Rico Association for Retarded
Citizens, Inc.
G.P.O. Box 1904
San Juan, PR 00936
809/764-5836
Contact: Carmen Lacomba

Puerto Rico Chapter of the Easter
Seal Society
G.P.O. Box 325
San Juan, PR 00936
809/767-6718
Contact: Roxanna De Soto,
Executive Director

RHODE ISLAND

Special Education Unit
Department of Education
Roger Williams Bldg., Rm. 200
22 Hayes St.
Providence, RI 02908
401/277-3505
Contact: Robert M. Pryhoda,
   Director

Department of Mental Health
Retardation & Hospitals
600 New London Ave.
Cranston, RI 02920
401/464-3201
Contact: Thomas Romeo, Director

Rhode Island P&A System, Inc.
86 Weybosset St., Suite 508
Providence, RI 02903
401/831-3150
Contact: Elizabeth Morancy,
   Executive Director

Association for Children with
   Learning Disabilities
P.O. Box 6685
Providence, RI 02904
401/274-7026
Contact: Cynthia Braca, Executive
   President

Mental Health Association
89 Park St.
Providence, RI 02908
401/272-6730
Contact: Susan M. Saunders,
   Executive Director

Association for Retarded Citizens
Craik Bldg.
2845 Post Rd.
Warwick, RI 02886
401/738-5550
Contact: James Healey, Executive
   Director

Easter Seal Society of Rhode Island
667 Waterman Avenue
East Providence, RI 02914
401/438-9500
Contact: Nancy B. D'Wolf, Executive
   Director

SOUTH CAROLINA

Office of Programs for the
   Handicapped
Koger Executive Center
100 Executive Center Dr.
Santee Bldg, Suite A-24
Columbia, SC 29210
803/737-8710
Contact: Robert S. Black, Ph.D.,
   Director

Superintendent of Special Programs
Department of Education Rutledge
   Building
Room 912-B
Columbia, SC 29201
803/734-8451
Contact: Annie Winstead, Ph.D.

Developmental Disabilities Council
1205 Pendleton St., Rm. 404
Columbia, SC 29201
803/758-8016
Contact: Dr. Sherry H. Driggers,
   Director

SC P&A System for the
Handicapped, Inc.
803/254–1600
1–800/922–5225
Contact: Louise Ravenel, Executive
Director

Epilepsy Association of South
Carolina
Columbia, SC
803/799–8341

Association for Children with
Learning Disabilities
414 Gentry St.
Spartanburg, SC 29303
803/573–8554
Contact: Lib Flowe, President

Association for Mental Health
1823 Gadsen Street
Columbia, SC 29201
803/779–5363
Contact: Donald Weyl, Executive
Director

South Carolina Association for
Retarded Citizens
7412 Fairfield Rd.
Columbia, SC 29202
803/754–4763
Contact: Dr. John E. Beckley,
Executive Director

SOUTH DAKOTA

Section for Special Education
Division of Education
700 N. Illinois St.
Pierre, SD 57501-2293
605/773–3315
Contact: Dr. George R. Levin,
Director

Secretary, Department of Vocational
Rehabilitation
700 N. Illinois St.
Pierre, SD 57501
605/773–3125
Contact: Mr. John E. Madigan

Office of Developmental Disabilities
and Mental Health
Department of Social Services
700 N. Illinois St.
Pierre, SD 57501
605/773–3438
Contact: Thomas E. Scheinost,
Director

Representative for Children
Office of Developmental Disabilities
and Mental Health
Department of Social Services
700 N. Illinois St.
Pierre, SD 57501
605/773–3438
Contact: Dianne Weyer

South Dakota Advocacy Project, Inc.
221 S. Central Avenue
Pierre, SD 57501
605/224–8294
800/742–8108
Contact: Robert J. Kean, Executive
Director

South Dakota Association for
Children with Learning Disabilities
1021 Fulton St.
Rapid City, SD 57105
605/342–0764
Contact: Jeanie Montgomery,
President

South Dakota Association for
  Retarded Citizens
222 W. Pleasant Drive
P.O. Box 502
Pierre, SD 57501
605/224-8211
Contact: John Stengle, Executive
  Director

Easter Seal Society of South Dakota
106 W. Capitol
Pierre, SD 57501
605/224-5879
Contact: Bart Bailey, Executive
  Director

South Dakota Parent Connection
4200 S. Louis St., Suite 205
Sioux Falls, SD 57106
605/361-0952
Contact: Judie Roberts

TENNESSEE

Division of Special Programs
132 Cordell Hull Bldg.
Nashville, TN 37219
615/741-2851
Contact: Dr. Joleta Reynolds,
  Assistant Commissioner

Special Vocational Programs
205 Cordell Hull Bldg.
Nashville, TN 37219
615/741-3446
Contact: Mr. Sam McClanahan,
  Specialist

Developmental Disabilities Council
James K. Polk Bldg., 4th Fl.
Nashville, TN 37219-5393
615/741-1742
Contact: Pat Oates, Director

Effective Advocacy for Citizens with
  Handicaps, Inc.
P.O. Box 121257
Nashville, TN 37212
615/298-1080
1-800/342-1660
Contact: Harriette Derryberry,
  Executive Director

Epilepsy Foundation of West
  Tennessee
Memphis, TN
901/452-7144

Epilepsy Foundation of Greater
  Chattanooga
Chattanooga, TN
615/756-1771

Epilepsy Foundation of Greater
  Knoxville
Knoxville, TN
615/524-8251

Epilepsy Foundation of Middle
  Tennessee
Nashville, TN
615/322-3322

Tennessee Association for Children
  with Learning Disabilities
P.O. Box 281028
Memphis, TN 38128
901/323-1430
Contact: Shera Bie, Executive
  Director

Mental Health Association of
  Tennessee
2416 Hillsboro Road
Nashville, TN 37212
615/298-1126
Contact: Faye Isaacs, Executive
  Secretary

Tennessee Association for Retarded
  Citizens
1700 Hayes St., Suite 200
Nashville, TN 37203
615/327–0294
Contact: Roger Blue, Executive
  Director

Easter Seal Society of Tennessee
2001 Woodmont Blvd.
P.O. Box 158145
Nashville, TN 37215
615/292–6639
1–800/423–9659

TEXAS

Special Education Program
William B. Travis Building
1701 N. Congress Avenue
Austin, TX 78701
512/463–9414
Contact: Jill Gray, Director

William B. Travis Building
1701 N. Congress Avenue
Austin, TX 78701
512/463–9446
Contact: Eleanor K. Mikulin,
  Occupational, Education Specialist
  for Special Needs

Texas Planning Council for the
  Developmentally Disabled
118 E. Riverside Dr.
Austin, TX 78704
512/445–8867
Contact: Roger A. Webb, Executive
  Director

Advocacy, Inc.
7700 Chevy Chase Dr., Ste. 300
Austin, TX 78752
512/454–4816
800/252–9108
Contact: Dayle Bebee, Executive
  Director

Ft. Worth/Tarrant County Epilepsy
  Association
Ft. Worth, TX
817/336–8693

Epilepsy Foundation of the
  Bluebonnet Region
San Antonio, TX
512/225–4540

Epilepsy Association of Houston/Gulf
  Coast
Houston, TX
713/861–1908

Texas Association for Children &
  Adults with Learning Disabilities
1011 w. 31st Street
Austin, TX 78705
512/458–8234
Contact: Dorothy Strance, Executive
  Director

Mental Health Association in Texas
117 W. 24th Street
Austin, TX 78705
512/476–0611
Contact: Stella Mullins, Executive
  Director

Association for Retarded Citizens,
  Texas
833 Houston Street
Austin, TX 78756
512/454-6694
Contact: Carmen Quesada,
  Executive Director

Texas Easter Seal Society
4300 Beltway Drive
Dallas, TX 75244
214/934-9104
Contact: Adele Foschia, Executive
  Director

UTAH

Special Education Section
State Office of Education
250 E. 5th South
Salt Lake City, UT 84111
801/533-5982
Contact: R. Elwood Pace, Director

Vocational Education for
  Disadvantaged and Handicapped
  Students
State Office for Vocational Education
250 East 500 South
Salt Lake City, UT 84111
801/533-5574
Contact: Kenneth L. Hennefer,
  Special Needs Coordinator

Utah Council for Handicapped and
  Developmentally Disabled Persons
P.O. Box 11356
Salt Lake City, UT 84147
801/533-6770
Contact: Frances Morse, Executive
  Director

Legal Center for the Handicapped
254 West 400 South, Suite 300
Salt Lake City, UT 84101
801/363-1347
1-800/662-9080
Contact: Phyllis Geldzahler,
  Executive Director

Epilepsy Association of Utah
Salt Lake City, UT
801/534-0210

Utah Association for Children with
  Learning Disabilities
5699 Wilderland Lane
Salt Lake City, UT 84118
801/967-0087
Contact: Carol Johanson, President

Mental Health Association of Utah
982 East 3300 South
Salt Lake City, UT 84106
801/486-4312
Contact: Alosia Carlson, President

Association for Retarded Citizens -
  Utah
455 E. 400 South, Suite 300
Salt Lake City, UT 84111
801/364-5060
1-800/662-4058
Contact: Ray Behle, Executive
  Director

Easter Seal Society of Utah
331 So. Rio Grande, Suite 206
Salt Lake City, UT 84101
801/531-0522
Contact: Lynn Jacobsen, Executive
  Director

Utah Parent Information and Training
  Center
4984 South 300 West
Murray, UT 84107
801/265-9883
1-800/468-1160
Contact: Jean E. Nash, Director

Utah Society for Children with
  Emotional Disabilities
6063 Sanford Drive
Murray, UT 84123
Contact: Diana Madsen, President

VERMONT

Special Education Unit
Department of Education
120 State St.
Montpelier, VT 05602
802/828-3141
Contact: Marc E. Hull, Ph.D., Chief

Vocational Education for
  Disadvantaged & Handicapped
  Programs
Department of Education
120 State St.
Montpelier, VT 05602
802/828-3101
Contact: Scott Davis, Special Needs
  Consultant

Vermont Developmentally Disabled
  Council
103 S. Main St.
Waterbury, VT 05676
802/241-2612
Contact: Thomas Pombar

Vermont Developmentally Disabled
  Law Project
6 Pine St.
Burlington, VT 05401
802/863-2881
Contact: William J. Reedy, Director

Epilepsy Association of Vermont
Rutland, VT
802/775-1686

Association for Children with
  Learning Disabilities
9 Heaton St.
Montpelier, VT 05602
802/223-5480

Vermont Association for Retarded
  Citizens
Champlain Mill, #37
Winooski, VT 05404
802/655-4014
Contact: Joan Sylvester, Executive
  Director

VIRGINIA

Department of Education
Disadvantaged/Handicapped
P.O. Box 6-Q
Richmond, VA 23216-2060
804/225-2402
Contact: William L. Helton, Ph.D.,
  Administrative Director for Special
  Education & Professional
  Development

Disadvantaged/Handicapped
Special Programs
Department of Education
P.O. Box 60
Richmond, VA 23216
804/225-2080
Contact: Vance Horne, Supervisor

Department of Mental Health &
  Mental Retardation
P.O. Box 1797
Richmond, VA 23214
804/786–5313
Contact: Linda Veldheer, Director of
  Developmental Disabilities

Department for Rights of the
  Disabled
James Monroe Bldg.
101 N. 14th St., 17th Fl.
Richmond, VA 23219
804/225–2042
1–800/552–3962
Contact: Carolyn White Hodgins,
  Director

Epilepsy Association of Virginia
Charlottesville, VA
804/924–5401

Learning Disabilities Council
P.O. Box 8451
Richmond, VA 23226
804/744–5177
Contact: Linda Williams, Executive
  Director

Mental Health Association
1806 Chantilly St., Suite 203
Richmond, VA 23230
804/353–2791
Contact: David E. Phillips, Jr.

Association of Retarded
  Citizens-Virginia
6 North 6th St., Suite 102
Richmond, VA 23219
804/649–8481

Easter Seal Society of Virginia, Inc.
4841 Williamson Rd.
P.O. Box 5496
Roanoke, VA 24012
703/362–1656
Contact: F. Robert Knight, Executive
  Director

Parent Educational Advocacy
  Training Center
228 South Pitt Street, Rm. 300
Alexandria, VA 22314
703/836–2953
Contact: Winifred Anderson, Director

WASHINGTON

Superintendent of Public Instruction
Old Capitol Bldg., F-G 11
Olympia, WA 98504
206/753–6733
Contact: Greg Kirsch, Director of
  Special Education

Developmental Disabilities Planning
  Council
Mail Stop GH-52
Olympia, WA 98504
206/753–3908
Contact: Sharon Hansen, Executive
  Director

The Troubleshooters Office
1550 West Armory Way, Suite 204
Seattle, WA 98119
206/284–1037
Contact: Katie Dolan, Executive
  Director

Epilepsy Association of W.
  Washington
Seattle, WA
206/523–2551

Washington Association for Children
with Learning Disabilities
300 120th Ave. NE
Bldg. 1, Suite 217
Bellvue, WA 98005
206/451-9171
Contact: L. Jones, Executive Director

Learning Disabilities Hotline
P.O. Box 46188
Seattle, WA 98146-0188
206/932-5507
Contact: Deborah Dishman

Washington Coalition for the
Mentally Ill
225 N. 70th St.
Seattle, WA 98103
206/789-7722
Contact: Eleanor Owen, Executive
Director

Washington Association for Retarded
Citizens
1703 E. State Ave.
Olympia, WA 98506
206/357-5596
Contact: James Marick, President

Easter Seal Society for Crippled
Children & Adults of Washington
521 Second Avenue, West
Seattle, WA 98119
206/281-5700
Contact: William E. Hunti, Executive
Director

Parents Advocating Vocational
Education - PAVE
1010 South Eye St.
Tacoma, WA 98406
206/272-7804

Parent/Community Relations Project
4160 86th Ave., SE
Mercer Island, WA 98040
206/233-3396
Contact: Martha Gentili, Director

Special Education Coalition
Parent Advisory Council Training
1703 E. State St.
Olympia, WA 98506
206/357-5596
Contact: Laila Adams, Director

WEST VIRGINIA

Office of Special Education
Administration
Capitol Complex
Bldg. 6, Room B-309
Charleston, WV 25305
304/348-7017
1-800/642-8541
Contact: William L. Capehart,
Director

Disadvantaged, Handicapped and
Work-Study Programs
State Department of Education
1900 Washington St.
Charleston, WV 25305
304/348-2349
Contact: Jean Cary Davis, Supervisor

Developmental Disabilities Planning
Council
1800 Washington St.
Charleston, WV 25305
304/348-2276
Contact: Richard Kelly, Director

West Virginia Advocates for the
Developmentally Disabled, Inc.
1200 Quarrier Street, Suite 27
Charleston, WV 25301
304/346-0847
1-800/642-9205
Contact: Nancy Mattox, Executive
Director

West Virginia Association for
Children with Learning Disabilities
1725 Crestmont Drive
Huntington, WV 25701
304/529-4985
Contact: Litz S. Jarvis

West Virginia Association for Mental
Health
702 1/2 Lee Street
Charleston, WV 25321
304/346-6005
Contact: Dorothy Whitehurst,
Executive Director

Association for Retarded Citizens in
WV
700 Market St.
Union Trust Bldg., Rm. 400
Parkersburg, WV 26101
304/485-5283

Easter Seal Society of West Virginia
1210 Virginia Street, East
Charleston, WV 25301
304/346-3508
Contact: John Stepp, Executive
Director

WISCONSIN

Division for Handicapped Children
and Pupil Services
125 S. Webster Street
P.O. Box 7841
Madison, WI 53707
608/266-1649
Contact: Victor Contrucci, State
Director

Vocational Special Needs Programs
Bureau for Vocational Education
Department of Public Instruction
125 S. Webster St., P.O. Box 7841
Madison, WI 53707
608/266-7987
Contact: Preston Smeltzer,
Supervisor

Wisconsin Council on
Developmental Disabilities
P.O. Box 7851
Madison, WI 53707
608/266-7826
Contact: Jayne Wittenmyer,
Executive Director

Wisconsin Coalition for Advocacy,
Inc.
16 N. Carroll, Suite 400
Madison, WI 53703-2716
608/251-9600
Contact: Lynn Breedlove, Executive
Director

Midstate Epilepsy Association
Stevens Point, WI
715/341-5811

Epilepsy Center-South Central
Madison, WI
608/257-5759

Wisconsin Epilepsy Association
Madison, WI
608/221-1210

Blackhawk Epilepsy Association
Janesville, WI
608/755-1821

Epilepsy Center of Western WI
Eau Claire, WI
715/834-4455

Wisconsin Association for Children
  with Learning Disabilities
2114 Doemel St.
Oshkosh, WI 54901
414/233-1977
Contact: John Burr, President

Mental Health Association of
  Wisconsin
119 East Mifflin Street
Madison, WI 53703
608/256-9041

Association for Retarded Citizens
5522 University Avenue
Madison, WI 53705
608/231-3335
Contact: Merlen Kurth, Executive
  Director

Easter Seal Society of Wisconsin, Inc.
2702 Monroe Street
Madison, WI 53711
608/231-3411
Contact: Roy Campbell, Executive
  Director

Parent Education Project
PEP Coalition/UCP of Southeastern
  Wisconsin, Inc.
152 W. Wisconsin Avenue
Milwaukee, WI 53202
414/272-4500
1-800/472-5525
Contact: Liz Irwin, Director

WYOMING

Special Programs Unit
State Department of Education
Hathaway Office Building
Cheyenne, WY 82002
307/777-7417
Contact: Kenneth A. Blackburn,
  Director

Special Needs Programs
State Department of Education
Hathaway Office Building
Cheyenne, WY 82002
307/777-6240
Contact: Renae Humburg,
  Vocational Education Consultant

State Planning Council on
  Developmental Disabilities
P.O. Box 265
21 Capitol Ave., Rm #505
ANB Building
Cheyenne, WY 82003
307/632-0775
Contact: Sharron Kelsey, Executive
  Director

Developmentally Disabled P&A
  System, Inc.
2424 Pioneer Avenue, Suite 101
Cheyenne, WY 82001
307/632-3496
Contact: Jeanne A. Kawcak,
  Executive Director

INDEX